Coping with Uncertainty: *Behavioral and Developmental Perspectives*

The Penn State Series On Child & Adolescent Development

Series Editors:
David S. Palermo and Richard M. Lerner

Palermo • Coping with Uncertainty: Behavioral and Developmental Perspectives

Coping with Uncertainty: *Behavioral and Developmental Perspectives*

Edited by
David S. Palermo
The Pennsylvania State University

LEA LAWRENCE ERLBAUM ASSOCIATES, PUBLISHERS
1989 Hillsdale, New Jersey Hove and London

Lawrence Erlbaum Associates, Inc., Pubishers
365 Broadway
Hillsdale, New Jersey 07642

Library of Congress Cataloging-in-Publication Data

Coping with uncertainty.

Based on a conference held at the Penn State campus, Oct. 30-Nov. 1, 1986; sponsored by the Foundation for Child Development.
Includes index.
1. Stress (physiology)—Congresses.
2. Uncertainty—Psychological aspects—Congresses.
3. Developmental psycobiology—Congresses.
I. Palermo, David Stuart, 1929- . II. Foundation for Child Development. [DNLM: 1. Adaptation, Physiological—congresses. 2. Adaptation, Psychological—congresses. 3. Human Development—congresses.
4. Stress, Psycological—congresses. WM 172 C7835 1986]
QP82.2.S8C66 1989 155 88-21448
ISBN 0-8058-0157-X

Printed in the United States of America
10 9 8 7 6 5 4 3 2 1

Contents

Contributors

Dr. David Blizard
Bowman-Gray School of Medicine
300 S. Hawthorne Road
Winston-Salem, NC 27013

John L. Beard
Department of Nutrition
The Pennsylvania State University
University Park, PA 16802

Dr. George P. Chrousos
NICHD
Building 10, 10 North
9000 Rockville Pike
Bethesda, MD 20205

Ms. Lorah Dorn
E-203 Henderson Building
The Pennsylvania State University
University Park, PA 16802

Dr. Robert O. Fisch
Department of Pediatrics
4125 Philip Wangensteen Building
University of Minnesota
Minneapolis, MN 55455

Dr. Philip W. Gold
Room 3S239, Bldg. 10
NIMH
9000 Rockville Park
Bethesda, MD 20205

Dr. Jeffrey Gray
Maudsley Hospital
De Grespigny Park
Denmark Hill
London, SE5 8AF
ENGLAND

Dr. Megan Gunnar
Institute of Child Development
University of Minnesota
51 East River Road
Minneapolis MN 55455

Dr. Joanna Hill
Sectionon Brain Biochemistry
Clinical Neuroscience Branch
NIMH, Building 10, Room 3N256
9000 Rockville Pike
Bethesda, MD

Dr. Jill Isensee
19361 Normandale
Prior Lake, MN 55372

Dr. Jerome Kagan
William James Hall
Harvard University
Cambridge, MA 02138

Diane R. Krieger, M.D.
Harvard Medical School
Beth Israel Hospital
Division of Endocrinology
and Metabolism
330 Brookline Avenue
Boston, MA 02215

Dr. Lewis Landsberg
Harvard Medical Schol
Beth Israel Hospital
Division of Endocrinology
and Metabolism
330 Brookline Avenue
Boston, MA 02215

Dr. Seymour Levine
Department of Psychiatry
and Behavioral Sciences
Primate Facility 7-930T
Stanford University
Stanford, CA 94305

Ms. Denny Marvinney
Indiana University
Psychology Clinic
Bloomington, IN 47401

Dr. Editha D. Nottelmann
Lab. of Developmental Psychology
NIMH
9000 Rockville Pike
Bethesda, MD 20205

Dr. Anne C. Petersen
Dean, College of Health
and Human Development
104 Henderson Building
The Pennsylvania State University
University Park, PA 16802

Dr. J. Steven Reznick
Department of Psychology
and Social Relations
Harvard University
33 Kirkland Street
Cambridge, MA 02138

Dr. Nancy Snidman
Department of Psychology
and Social Relations
Harvard University
33 Kirkland Street
Cambridge, MA 02138

Dr. Elizabeth J. Susman
E-203 Henderson Building
The Pennsylvania State University
University Park, PA 16802

Dr. Sandra G. Wiener
Department of Psychiatry
Stanford University School
of Medicine
Stanford University
Stanford, CA 94305-5095

Preface

This book marks the beginning of a new series growing out of the activities of The Center for the Study of Child and Adolescent Development at The Pennsylvania State University. In a sense, this volume provides a scholarly tribute to the vision of Dean Evan G. Pattishall, Jr. He recognized the large body of individuals interested in developmental processes spread across the Penn State campus and suggested the formation of a Center that would act to coalesce that group for their benefit and, in so doing, bring about the formation of a nucleus of individuals who might have a significant impact on our understanding of the developmental processes. Thus, in 1984, the Center came into being. Richard Lerner was appointed as director and I accepted the position as associate director. Among the many activities we initiated as a part of achieving the goals we set for the Center was the initiation of a series of conferences that focus on the most important developing ideas in the field.

As the first meeting of our Advisory Board, convened for the purposes of guiding the early activities of the Center, we discussed our conference plans and Jerry Kagan indicated that he had been thinking of a conference concerned with the physiology and psychology of stress. The idea had several attractive features. First, the focus of the conference had obvious developmental implications that had received little attention from those working in these areas. Second, the problem was interdisciplinary, a natural aspect of our conception of the Center. Thus, with Jerry's help we selected and invited an outstanding group of researchers drawn from those who have approached the problem from the physiological and/or the psychological side of the issue. We asked them to discuss the relations between the biological stress circuits—including the pituitary–adrenal axis, the reticular activating system, and the autonomic nervous system—and the behavioral concomitants to stress in animals and humans. In addition, we asked the participants to think and talk about the developmental implications of their work in relation to the periods of infancy, childhood, and adolescence, a task some found challenging.

The conference was held on the Penn State campus, October 30 to November 1, 1986. The persons in attendance who made presentations were Seymore Levine, Joanna M. Hill, Jeffrey Gray, David A. Blizard, Stephen J. Suomi, George P. Chrousos, Phillip W. Gold, Jerome Kagan, Megan R. Gunnar, Anne C. Petersen, Elizabeth J. Susman, Lewis Landsberg, and Gerald McClearn. In addition to the audience of persons from Penn State and surrounding areas, we were pleased to have as invited participant–observers Ilan Baruch, Nathan A. Fox, J. D. Higley, Denny Marvinney, and G.S. Pauley. The chapters in this book reflect the revisions of the papers given at that conference taking into consideration some of the insightful comments made by others at the meeting itself.

We are grateful to the Foundation for Child Development which supported the Center in sponsoring the conference.

David S. Palermo

1

Coping With Uncertainty: *A Paradox*

Seymour Levine
Sandra G. Wiener
Stanford University School of Medicine

When one examines the subject matter of this volume, coping with uncertainty, there is an initial intuitive gestalt. When one attempts to define the concepts and to discuss them in terms of available theoretical and scientific information, a world of confusing definitions is entered. There appear to be two basic approaches to the concept of coping. The first approach is probably best illustrated by the research of Lazarus (Lazarus, 1966). He proposed a classification of coping based on whether the function of the coping response is to alter the disturbed person–environment interaction or to regulate emotion. Another classification is based on the coping mode that is utilized. Coping modes are classified into information seeking, direct action, inhibition of action, and various interpsychic modes. These classifications are somewhat diffuse and it is not altogether certain whether they reflect dimensions that relate in any way to outcome. Lazarus, Averill, and Opton (1974) defined *coping* as follows: "Coping involves problem solving efforts made by an individual when the demands he faces are highly relevant to his welfare, that is, a situation of considerable jeopardy or promise, and when these demands tax his adaptive resources" (pp. 250–251). Such a definition does several things: First, it emphasizes the importance of the emotional context in coping; second, it allows inclusion of both a negative or stress side of emotions, as well as a positive side of potential fulfillment or gratification; third, it recognizes the overlap between problem solving and coping; and fourth, it emphasizes tasks that are not routine or automatized, that is, those in which the outcomes are uncertain and in which the limits of the individual's adaptive skills are approached.

What is clear from the definition proposed by Lazarus is that some coping processes may increase the risk of maladaptive behaviors, whereas others may improve adaptation and reduce the risk of a negative outcome. Thus, there exists a distinction between effective and ineffective coping within Lazarus' concept of coping. It appears that there is not one successful coping strategy. The coping mode that might be most effective is likely to be dependent on the type of stress and the context in which the stress occurs. Further, there may be clearly idiosyncratic approaches in the coping mode that is utilized. Central to the definition of coping used by Lazarus is the concept that an individual's cognitive appraisal of the stressful event strongly determines his or her responses (Lazarus & Launier, 1978). The same event may be perceived by different individuals as threatening and harmful or as benign and positive. Further, Lazarus and Launier have theorized that there is another appraisal process (secondary appraisal) that deals with an individual's conceptualization of the implications of the events in terms of coping resources and options. Thus, from this perspective, coping with uncertainty would involve one or multiple strategies, mostly cognitive, which would determine the ultimate failure or success of the coping strategy.

It appears that coping has been evaluated in at least two ways: One, a judgment is made as to whether a behavior allows the individual to execute certain personally and socially defined goals and to tolerate the stress of the situation without disruptive anxiety or depression, regardless of whether the behavior is socially desirable. Second, alterations in internal states can be evaluated by monitoring changes in physiological responses. One example is that cortisol excretion rates appear to be stable if coping behavior is effective in protecting the individual from anxiety and depression (Friedman, Mason, & Hamburg, 1963). It should be noted that both pathological and/or socially desirable coping patterns can affect these changes.

There is, however, a second approach to the coping process that was first elaborated by the now classic experiments of stress-induced stomach ulceration by Weiss (1972). Perhaps the primary difference between the concepts developed by Weiss and those espoused by Lazarus is that in the Weiss theory there can be no unsuccessful coping. Coping is therefore defined by a positive outcome that for the most part is based on reduction of pathological or physiological indices. For example, the organism is presumed to be coping if it has either reduced or eliminated stomach ulceration as a consequence of specific environmental contingencies. In addition to stomach ulcerations, other physiological indices of stress (e.g., endocrine, autonomic, neurophysiological, and immunological measures) have been demonstrated to be modulated either in terms of being significantly reduced or, in some instances, being eliminated as a consequence of specific behavioral or other clearly specified environmental events.

This second approach to coping was developed by examining the effects of psychological variables in stressful situations. The general procedure consists of exposing two or more animals to the same physical stressor while maintaining the subjects in different psychological conditions. When this is done, any difference that results from treatments must be attributed to psychological differences between the conditions because the physical stressor is measurably the same. It appears that psychological factors are often far more critical in influencing certain outcomes than the physical stimuli themselves, even if the stimuli are intensely noxious. Psychological variables that have been studied most often are those related to controllability, feedback, and predictability of stress. The ability to perform appropriate responses during stress and the previous experience of the organism in relation to these factors are critical factors in coping.

Insofar as there have been detailed descriptions and discussion of the coping mechanisms proposed by Weiss (1972), they are only described briefly here. *Control* can best be defined as the capacity to make active responses during the presence of an aversive stimulus. *Responses* are effective in permitting the organism to either avoid or escape the stimulus, but they also permit the animal the opportunity to alter one set of stimulus conditions to another. *Feedback* is defined as information after the response. These stimuli appear to have the capacity to impart information to the responding animal, indicating that it has performed correctly, or that it has terminated the aversive stimuli. Although it has been reported that *predictability* of stimuli tend to reduce these somatic reactions when compared to organisms receiving unpredictable aversive events, the effects of predictability are less clear cut. An analysis of the consequences of predictability are presented by Weinberg and Levine (1980).

It is proposed that the intensity of stress that an organism encounters when exposed to noxious stimuli is dependent on two factors: the number of coping attempts made by the animal and the amount of relevant feedback. As the number of coping attempts increases and the amount of relevant feedback decreases there is a marked increase in the stress response. Numerous studies have demonstrated that if two groups of subjects were exposed to the same shock, the pathological consequences of the shock were ameliorated if the animal could control the duration of shock and/or the situation was signaled by either a warning signal preceding the shock or a feedback signal following shock (Weiss, 1971a, 1971b, 1971c).

A close examination of the three major variables—control, predictability, and feedback—indicate that they have common elements that can be viewed as having the capacity to reduce uncertainty. Control provides the organism with the capacity to eliminate or at least to regulate the duration and/or intensity of the stimuli. Thus, the uncertainty involved in an unpredictable and uncontrollable situation would be reduced by control. Predictability, by definition, serves to reduce uncertainty. Feedback can also be viewed in terms of reducing uncertainty because feedback provides information to the organism about the efficacy and success of the response being emitted. We can therefore speculate that cognitive and behavioral processes that reduce uncertainty result in a reduction or elimination of one or more physiological responses to a stressful situation. Thus, elimination or reduction of adverse physiological events is what can be defined as *coping*.

In an extensive analysis of the psychological factors that regulate one of the major stress-responding systems, the hypothalamic-pituitary-adrenal (HPA) axis, it has been hypothesized that neuroendocrine activation of this system can best be described as a response to uncertainty (Hennessy & Levine, 1979). In the analysis of psychological factors that regulate the HPA system one cannot avoid making reference to cognitive processes. It is, again, unfortunate that the term *cognitive* is used in this context, because it creates some confusion with the cognitive processes described by Lazarus. Berlyne (1960, 1967) presented a theory of arousal that provides the framework for a description of the processes by which stimulators of arousal operate. Novelty, uncertainty, and conflict are considered arousing. These have been labeled by Berlyne as "collative" factors, because in order to evaluate them it is necessary to compare similarities and differences between stimulus elements (novelty) or between stimulus evoked expectations (uncertainty).

Hennessy and Levine (1979) have proposed that the responses of the HPA system are a reflection of changes in the level of the hypothetical construct of arousal. The approach taken was to demonstrate that the activation of the HPA system was subject to the same parametric relationships between stimulus and training variables as arousal. It would then follow that the basic cognitive processes involved in the regulation of the HPA system is one of comparison. The cognitive process of comparison can best be understood by invoking the concept of *uncertainty*.

Neuroendocrine activation in response to uncertainty relies heavily on the model elaborated by Sokolov (1960). Although Sokolov's model was one proposed to account for habituation, in fact, it appears to be a powerful explanatory concept with regard to understanding the arousal-inducing effects of uncertainty. Sokolov's model, in essence, is based on a matching system in which new stimuli or situations are compared with the representation in the central nervous system of prior events. This matching process results in development of expectancies whereby the organism is considered either habituated or, conversely, emits an alerting reaction to a mismatch (Pribram & Melges, 1969). If the environment does not contain any new stimuli or contingencies, the habituated organism no longer responds with a physiological response related to the alerting reaction. Thus, novelty, according to the theory of Sokolov, is one of the most potent variables that elicits an increase in HPA activity. Although novelty can be assumed under the general heading of uncertainty, not all conditions that create uncertainty are novel. Uncertainty can be evoked by insufficient information concerning the nature of upcoming events, and can be viewed to vary along a continuum of highly certain (predictable) to highly uncertain (unpredictable) events. The presentation of a novel stimulus is likely to lead to increased uncertainty because there is little information the organism can use to predict forthcoming events.

Uncertainty can also be defined in terms of contingencies between environmental events. Experimentally, the dimension of uncertainty can be influenced by limiting the amount of information available to the organism to predict the occurrence of a specific event. Thus, one would hypothesize that if an organism is given information about the occurrence of either an appetitive or aversive stimulus, such predictability would lead to a reduction in the HPA response. Further, in situations in which there is an absence of predictability, feedback or control would modulate physiological responses. The experimental evidence supporting the concept of uncertainty as a mediator of the response of the HPA system has been well documented (Hennessy & Levine, 1979; Levine, 1985; Levine, Goldman, & Coover, 1972). Uncertainty is the major determinant of inducing arousal responses that are clearly evident in a number of physiological systems but primarily in the HPA system, and those behavioral and environmental contingencies that serve to reduce uncertainty also serve to diminish or eliminate these responses. Thus, coping with uncertainty is a paradox, because by these criterion coping basically involves reduction of uncertainty.

It is not the purpose of this discussion to attempt to resolve the apparent differences between these two approaches to coping elaborated by Lazarus and Weiss. Some aspects of Lazarus' coping theory are very consistent with the approach taken by Weiss. Thus, coping modes, which consist of initiation of action or problem solving, can be easily subsumed under the general rubric of control. However, what cannot be dealt with is Lazarus' concept of inefficient coping. The problem is made even more difficult by the fact that the primary emphasis in the coping literature has been on behavioral responses in humans, whereas in the psychobiological literature, using both animals and humans, *coping* has been defined in terms of both the behavioral and physiological consequences. When there is consistency between behavioral changes and physiological changes it is simple to incorporate both into either definition of coping. However, there are numerous instances where behavioral and physiological indices of coping are dissociated. One such example is an experiment by Weinberg and Levine (1980), in which animals were trained in an active avoidance task. When the plasma corticoid response of nonlearners was compared to animals that had learned to avoid the shock, both types of animals showed a significant reduction of plasma corticoids following a period of training. Whereas nonlearning can be considered an inappropriate coping behavior, the same reduction in plasma corticoid occurred in both learners and nonlearners. This reduction in the physiological response was interpreted as indicating that although the nonlearners did not avoid the electric shock, they did escape, which terminated the conditioned stimulus (CS). This termination of the CS provided a sufficient feedback signal, which permitted a reduction of physiological arousal as measured by HPA activity.

Insofar as we are unable to resolve the differences between these theoretical approaches to coping, it becomes even more important to specify precisely what is being defined as coping within the context of this chapter. An extensive literature indicates that biological changes that occur under stress, if permitted to persist, can lead to pathological states (Munck, Guyre, & Holbrook, 1984). It appears that a reduction of the physiological response to aversive stimuli, whether or not appropriate behavior is emitted at that time, could be considered as relevant and adaptive changes for survival. Therefore, within the context of this chapter, we are defining *coping* as based on the reduction or elimination of the physiological responses produced as a consequence of uncertainty. This is clearly not a statement of truth, but a statement of preference.

COPING AND DEVELOPMENT

Insofar as this volume is dedicated primarily to developmental processes, it is important to translate the concepts of coping that we have discussed into a developmental perspective. This approach is hardly novel, as the importance of control has long been recognized as a salient feature in the ontogeny of coping. The infant's initial experience with contingency and control are, by definition, within the context of the mother–infant relationship. Lewis and Goldberg (1969) have stated that "Contingency is of importance, not only because it shapes the acquisition of certain behaviors, but because it enables the child to develop a motive which is the basis for all future learning. The main characteristic of this motive is the infant's belief that its actions affect his environment" (p. 82). The mother is important because it is the contingency between the infant's behavior and her responses that enables the infant to learn that its behavior has consequences. Mason (1978), in a discussion concerning the difference between infant rhesus that were raised with stationary surrogates and infant rhesus raised with dogs, commented:

> I believe that the critical distinction between attachment figures in these experiments is the presence or absence of response contingent stimulation. Stationary surrogates and hobby horses surely provide few opportunities for a developing individual to experience the fact that his behavior has effects on the environment and to learn that the events going on around him are amenable to his control. Inert mother substitutes make no demands, occasion no surprises, do not encourage the development of attentional processes and the acquisition of simple instrumental behaviors that are the fabric of social interactions. (p. 249)

It has been proposed, therefore, that these early contingent relationships are fundamental in order for the infant to learn certain cogent aspects of its environment that permit the infant to acquire adaptive coping responses. These early experiences with control appear to be essential in normal infant development and they also permit the infant to become an adaptive, functioning adult. In comparison, surrogate-reared infants raised in a noncontingent environment display many behavioral aberrations as adults.

It is now almost a decade since this laboratory published its first papers showing striking endocrine changes, particularly in the HPA system, associated with brief periods of separation in the infant squirrel monkey (Coe, Mendoza, Smotherman, & Levine, 1978; Levine, Coe, Smotherman, & Kaplan, 1978; Mendoza et al., 1978). Although we initially assumed that we were studying the psychobiological sequelae of disruptions in attachment, subsequent data obtained from behavioral and physiological measures (i.e., plasma cortisol and cerebrospinal fluid [CSF] monoamine metabolites) during separation have resulted in our interpreting these data more within the coping framework than the framework of attachment theory. This approach was dictated by the data that emerged from a series of studies that dealt with the various aspects of the separation environment. The results obtained while measuring behavioral and physiological responses simultaneously were unexpected and difficult to explain by attachment theory. We have found that the separation response is highly dependent on the conditions of separation, and there are many constraints on both behavioral and physiological responses that are determined by the environmental context during separation.

In our initial studies examining the HPA response to separation, it was found that the squirrel monkey infant displayed an increase in vocalization and a significant elevation in plasma cortisol levels when the infant was separated from its mother and placed in a novel cage totally isolated from other conspecifics for a 30-minute period. These data are consistent with the hypothesis that increased vocalization is a signal of distress in that the infant also showed a concomitant increase in plasma cortisol levels. This concordance of behavioral and physiological responses could be interpreted as indicating similar processes. However, this interpretation of the data was very rapidly demonstrated to be much too simple. As we extended the period of separation, we observed that squirrel monkey infants continued to show a progressive elevation of plasma cortisol, so that at 24 hours after separation the plasma cortisol values were approximately five times higher than those observed after a brief 30-minute separation (see Fig. 1.1). In contrast, vocalization rates declined during this period (see Fig. 1.2). Although the infants were not vocalizing 24 hours after separation, their behavior was not similar to the depression that has been reported for Old World monkeys following separation. The infants were active (e.g., eating, drinking, and exploring the environment) 24 hours following separation. In our laboratory, using both rhesus and infant squirrel monkeys, we have only on rare occasions seen anything that resembles a depressive response. This inverse relationship between vocalization and the physiological response to separation has been very consistent in numerous studies in our laboratory and can be

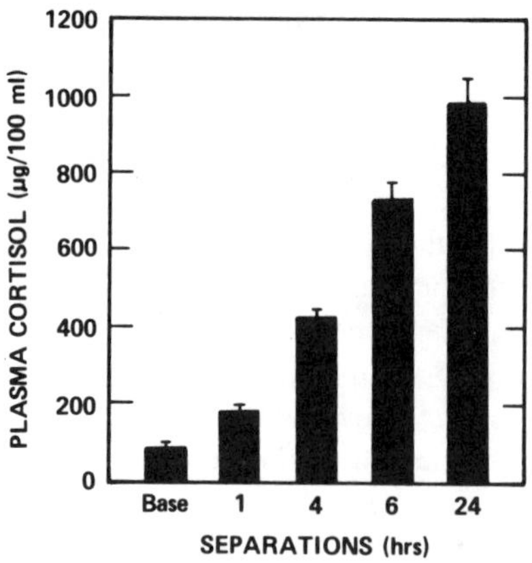

FIG. 1.1 Time course of the infant plasma cortisol (μg/100 ml response (SEM) to total isolation from the mother (Coe et al., 1985).

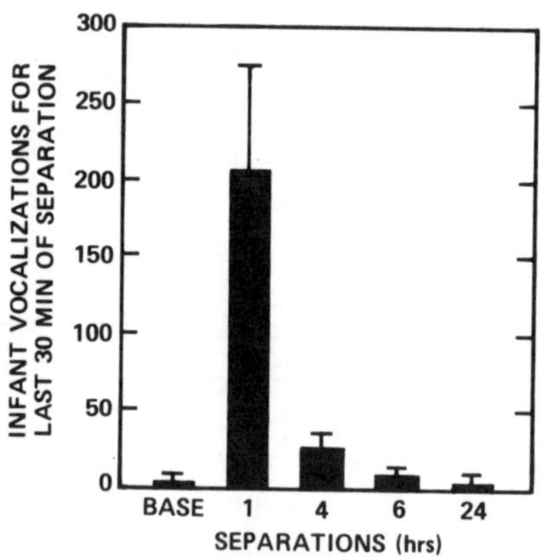

FIG. 1.2 Time course of the infant vocalizations ($\overline{x} \pm$ SEM) emitted to total isolation during the last 30 minutes of separation (Levine et al., 1978).

illustrated by the following studies, which have manipulated the separation environment into which the infant is placed.

Under normal circumstances, it is the proximity and contact with the mother that modulates and reduces the infant's stress responses (Coe, Wiener, Rosenberg, & Levine, 1985). The aversiveness of involuntary separation is due not only to loss of the mother but also to exposure to an unfamiliar environment. Vocalizations, in particular the isolation call, emitted by the infant are the primary means through which the primate infant elicits caregiving behavior. The infant has had extensive experience with the efficacy of calling since birth. Thus, it is not surprising that separation initially evokes a high level of calls. However, the absence of the usual reinforcer for this response, the mother, results in a rapid cessation of calling. We have also observed that following six 1-hour separations, calling was significantly reduced, whereas there is no reduction in the plasma cortisol response to separation (Coe, Glass, Wiener, & Levine, 1983). The plasma cortisol response to separation is highly persistent. In one study by Jordan et al. (1984), it was demonstrated that plasma cortisol responses were elevated following 20 separations, and Hennessy (1986) has reported that the adrenal response persists even after 80 daily separations.

One of the variables that has been shown to affect the behavioral response following separation is the degree of access the infant has to the mother during the separation period. Infants separated from mothers by wire mesh partition, which allowed minimal physical contact, showed only a very small degree of so-called distress behaviors. However, when the members of the dyad were separated by a Plexiglas panel, which prevented tactile contact, the usual infant protest behavior was observed (Suomi, Collins, Harlow, & Ruppenthal, 1976). Seay and Harlow (1965) reported that infants with no access to the mother (removed to a separate area) exhibited less protest behavior (vocalizations) than infants separated from the mother by Plexiglas. We have also demonstrated that rhesus infants, totally isolated from the mother and other conspecifics, emitted less vocalization than those infants separated in view of their mothers or social group (Levine, Franklin, & Gonzales, 1984). Because most of the initial research relied heavily on vocalization as a measure of distress, it was concluded that exposure to the mother produced the greatest distress and that removal of the infant from the mother supported the "out-of-sight, out-of-mind" notion. In view of the reported inverse relationship between infant cortisol levels and vocalization rates, it can be argued that these vocalizations emitted early in separation, particularly when visual access to the mother is available, represent active coping attempts on the part of the infant. Thus, it would be predicted that the physiological indices of arousal would be reduced in infants making active coping attempts when separated in visual proximity to the mother. One would also predict that vocalizations would tend to persist at a higher level in those animals separated in visual proximity to the mother, because the cues that are required to elicit these coping responses would be continually available.

Initial experiments to test these hypotheses were conducted with rhesus macaques (Levine, 1987; Levine, Johnson, & Gonzales, 1985). Two experiments clearly support the hypothesis that visual access to the mother produced different behavioral responses and modulated the physiological response to separation. The basic paradigm for both of these experiments, although differing somewhat in detail, was to separate infants, either totally isolated from other monkeys or to separate them adjacent to the mother where visual and auditory cues were present, but contact was prevented. The findings demonstrated that visual access to the mother produced significantly higher levels of calling and significantly lower levels of plasma cortisol and the CSF metabolite of norepinephrine, MHPG, than the totally isolated infant. These data are consistent with our view that the most physiologically arousing situation appears to be total isolation that entails separation from the mother and from the social group simultaneously. Once again, behavioral and physiological responses appear to be not concordant. However, the hypothesis generated by coping theory would expect these events to be highly related. Under conditions of stress, proximity and contact with mother should result in a reduction of the infant's arousal levels and one of the primary behavioral responses that achieves proximity and contact in primates is vocalization. When cues of the mother are available, the infant should vocalize in an attempt to achieve proximity. Although proximity and contact are not possible under the condition of adjacent separation in this experiment, it appears that vocalization still serves to reduce arousal, which leads to either reduced or nonsignificant changes in the plasma cortisol response and reduced elevations of CSF MHPG levels.

Perhaps one of the most surprising findings in this series of rhesus separation experiments came when the vocalizations emitted by the infants during the total and adjacent separations were spectrographically analyzed. This analysis revealed that there were different types of calls made under the two conditions of separation. It appears that not only the number of calls emitted under the two separation conditions differed, but the information imparted by the calls may be significantly different.

A subsequent study was conducted using the squirrel monkey. The paradigm used was similar to that described earlier for rhesus macaques. In this experiment, we examined infant squirrel monkeys separated for 24 hours under three different conditions: (a) total isolation—infant removed from its mother and placed in a novel cage isolated from other monkeys; (b) adjacent—dyad removed from the social group and placed in adjacent cages that prevent physical contact; (c)home—mother removed from the social group and infant permitted to remain in the home social group composed of other mother–infant dyads. The rate of emitted vocalizations discriminated between these conditions of separation. Thus, under the home condition, where the infant is in the presence of familiar conspecifics, the amount of vocalization emitted was lowest. Under the adjacent condition, similar to that observed in rhesus monkeys, there were continued high levels of vocalization. In the total condition, vocalizations were significantly elevated for the first 30 minutes, but by 6 and 24 hours there were very few vocalizations. However, even when the vocalization rates were elevated under the total condition, the rates were significantly lower than those observed under adjacent separation. Thus, we have demonstrated that vocalization rates appear to be determined by the environmental conditions of separation with home and total isolation conditions yielding lower vocalizations than those observed under adjacent separation. The plasma cortisol of separated infants also indicated significant differences between each of the separation conditions. Infants separated from their mothers in the home social group displayed the lowest plasma cortisol elevation above base compared to either the total or adjacent conditions. Totally isolated infants displayed the greatest elevation in plasma cortisol levels and the infants adjacent to their mothers during separation displayed intermediate levels of plasma cortisol. Similarly, elevations of

CSF metabolites of norepinephrine (MHPG) and dopamine (HVA) discriminated between the adjacent and total conditions with the latter higher than the former.

The results of the aforementioned study would appear to only partially support the postulated inverse relationship between physiological arousal and vocalization. The high vocalization rate and low plasma cortisol in the adjacent condition and the low vocalization rate and high plasma cortisol in the total isolation condition are consistent with our model. However, there is an exception to this seemingly reliable inverse relationship between vocalization and HPA activity. This is observed when the infants are separated from their mother but permitted to remain in the home social group with familiar conspecifics; these infants displayed the lowest vocalization rates and the lowest elevation of plasma cortisol levels following separation. The familiar social environment is unique when compared to our other environmental conditions. It has been demonstrated that familiarity, per se, with separation environment is not relevant. Infants reared only with their mothers in individual cages did not exhibit reduced behavioral or physiological responses when left at home during separation (Wiener, Johnson, & Levine, 1987). Thus, the presence of familiar conspecifics appears to be the important factor in modulating the infant's physiological response to separation in this home condition.

In several other studies, using both infants and adult organisms, we have demonstrated that social interactions with other members of the group seems to be an important variable in modulating neuroendocrine activity when exposed to aversive stimuli (Coe, Franklin, Smith, & Levine, 1982; Stanton, Patterson, & Levine, 1985). It is possible to still use other aspects of the coping model to account for the effects of a familiar social group resulting in a reduction of both the behavioral and the physiological responses to separation. It is proposed that social interactions are also an important modulator of the response to separation, due primarily to the predictability of the social interactions with familiar conspecifics. Due to the long previous experience of interactions with familiar social partners, it appears that social partners have the capacity to buffer the response of both infants and adults to stress-inducing situations. The proposed mechanism for buffering this response may derive from the fact that the infant is in an environment where all previous social interactions are highly predictable and, therefore, the presence of these predictable relationships is what accounts for the modulation of the HPA activation following separation. In addition, it is possible that under these circumstances the infants have the opportunity to maintain contact and proximity with other familiar social partners. This contact and proximity, albeit not with the mother, may be capable of reducing the responses to the loss of the maternal figure.

It is important to emphasize that the conditions that suppress both plasma cortisol and vocalization following separation are ones in which the infant is in contact or proximity with *familiar* social partners. All aspects of the coping model would predict that the most intensely stressful condition would be when the infant experiences separation from the mother in the presence of unfamiliar conspecifics. The infant would not only be in a novel, arousing environment, but would further be exposed to a set of highly unpredictable social interactions that promotes even greater distress on the part of the infant. We have conducted one such study in which the infant was separated and placed with a strange social group during separation (Levine & Wiener, 1988). These infants exhibited almost immediate secession in vocalization and displayed the most elevated cortisol levels found in any of our studies in which the separation environment has been the manipulated variable.

In light of the large amount of data indicating an inverse relationship between the behavioral measures (i.e., vocalizations and activity) and the physiological indices of distress, it was necessary that we reinterpret the meaning of the behavioral data. Using a more functional view, we hypothesized that the results are more consistent with a stress and coping theory approach than the original basis for the research, the biology of attachment. Perhaps the most compelling reason for this view is the strong effect that environmental conditions have on the separation response. Although other investigators have previously reported environmental effects on the separation response in both human and animal studies (McGinnis, 1980; Mineka & Suomi, 1978; Robertson & Robertson, 1971; Weinraub & Lewis, 1977), the empirical data has not altered how most investigators interpret the infant's behavior after maternal separation. Rosenblum and Plimpton (1981) pointed out that most researchers continue to interpret the infant's response to loss as a ballistic model. This model follows an orderly progression of the affective response from the initial protest reaction to the subsequent depression and withdrawal. Discussions on the influence of the environment or prior experience, therefore, focus primarily on the occurrence and intensity of the depressive phase. Our data suggested to us instead that environmental and experiential factors exert an immediate influence on how the infant perceives the loss and on its behavioral options for dealing with separation. The infant's response is not simply reactive in an emotional sense, but reflects an active attempt to alter the aversive situation. Thus, we question the use of vocalization as an index of emotional disturbance. Alternately, we have proposed to evaluate this aspect of the behavioral response in coping terms.

CONCLUSIONS

Since the 1950s, numerous studies have been reported on the response of human and primate infants to separation and maternal loss. Initially, the research using nonhuman primates was concerned with establishing an experimental basis of attachment. Following Bowlby's (1969) review of these studies, investigators began to examine other aspects of the infant's response to maternal loss. As a consequence, we are now aware that the infant's response is not invariable and can be influenced by multiple factors that include the context within which separation occurs, prior experience of separation, and genetic variables. Studies have also demonstrated that there are numerous physiological changes that accompany the behavioral manifestations following separation (Coe & Levine, 1981; Kraemer & McKinney, 1979; Reite, Short, & Seiler, 1978). The research that emanated from the Laboratory of Developmental Psychobiology at Stanford has been concerned with the relationship between these physiological responses and the infant's behavioral reaction to separation. From the data obtained, we have attempted to apply many of the concepts elaborated in the literature of stress and coping to explain the relationship between behavioral and physiological changes following separation. It is our belief that this perspective offers a new approach in attempting to understand the relationship between infants' behavioral and physiological responses to separation. All of the early studies on mother–infant separations depended exclusively on behavioral measures to assess the infant's level of disturbance with major emphasis placed on vocalization and activity. When we first began our research, it was with the conviction that we would be able to infer internal physiological changes from external behavior.

We have shown that behavioral responses to separation are entirely dependent on the manner and conditions of separation and, therefore, do not necessarily relate positively with physiological responses. Further, it is often difficult to predict the degree of physiological activation from the intensity of the behavioral response. What has emerged is that by simultaneously assessing the behavioral and physiological responses following separation, we have been forced to reexamine both of these dimensions with regard to regulation and control. Within the framework of psychobiological investigations, the problem is not determining which of the particular parameters measured reflects the true process. The fact is that both reflect processes that are going on within the organism. What is important is that by having available information from two sources of the organism's response capacities, we are able to examine, and in this instance to reinterpret, the behaviors within another theoretical context.

To summarize, we believe that uncertainty is a potent activator of autonomic and endocrine activity. The primary function of the coping process, which includes control, feedback, and predictability, is to reduce uncertainty. For the developing infant, it appears that these coping processes occur within the context of contingent mother–infant relationships. It is within this context that the infant first learns that its behavior has consequences. These consequences appear to include the ability to utilize behaviors and environmental stimuli to reduce uncertainty.

ACKNOWLEDGMENTS

The research was supported by research grant HD-02881 from NICH&HD and a Career Research Scientist Award MH-19336 from NIMH to S. Levine.

REFERENCES

Berlyne, D. E. (1960). *Conflict, arousal and curiosity.* New York: McGraw–Hill.

Berlyne, D. E. (1967). Arousal and reinforcement. In D. Levine (Ed.), *Nebraska Symposium on Motivation* (pp. 1–110). Lincoln: University of Nebraska Press.

Bowlby, J. (1969). *Attachment and loss.* New York: Basic.

Coe, C. L., Franklin, D., Smith, E. R., & Levine, S. (1982). Hormonal responses accompanying fear and agitation in the squirrel monkey. *Physiology and Behavior, 29,* 1051–1057.

Coe, C. L., Glass, J. C., Wiener, S. G., & Levine, S. (1983). Behavioral, but not physiological, adaptation to repeated separation in mother and infant primates. *Psychoneuroendocrinology, 8,* 401–409.

Coe, C. L., & Levine, S. (1981). Normal responses to mother–infant separation in non–human primates. In D. F. Klein & J. G. Rabkin (Eds.), *Anxiety: New research and changing concepts* (pp. 155–177). New York: Raven.

Coe, C. L., Mendoza, S. P., Smotherman, W. P., & Levine, S. (1978). Mother-infant attachment in the squirrel monkey: Adrenal response to separation. *Behavioral Biology, 22,* 256–263.

Coe, C. L., Wiener, S. G., Rosenberg, L. T., & Levine, S. (1985). Physiological consequences of maternal separation and loss in the squirrel monkey. In L. A. Rosenblum & C. L. Coe (Eds.), *The handbook of squirrel monkey research* (pp. 127–148). New York: Plenum Press.

Friedman, S. B., Mason, J. W., & Hamburg, D. A. (1963). Urinary 17–hydroxycorticosteroid levels in parents of children with neoplastic disease: A study of chronic psychological stress. *Psychosomatic Medicine, 25,* 364–376.

Hennessy,J. W., & Levine, S. (1979). Stress, arousal, and the pituitary–adrenal system: A psychoendocrine hypothesis. In J. M. Sprague & A. N. Epstein (Eds.), *Progress in psychobiology and physiological psychology* (pp. 133–178). New York: Academic Press.

Hennessy, M. B. (1986). Multiple, brief maternal separations in the squirrel monkey: Changes in hormonal and behavioral responsiveness. *Physiology & Behavior, 36,* 245–250.

Jordan, T. C., Coe, C. L., Patterson, J., & Levine, S. (1984). Predictability and coping with separation in infant squirrel monkeys. *Behavioral Neuroscience, 98,* 556–560.

Kraemer, G. W., & McKinney, W. T. (1979). Interaction of pharmacological agents which alter biogenic amine metabolism and depression. *Journal of Affective Disorders, 1,* 33–54.

Lazarus, R. S. (1966). *Psychological stress and the coping process.* New York: McGraw–Hill.

Lazarus, R. S., Averill, J. R., & Opton, E. M., Jr. (1974). The psychology of coping: Issues of research and assessment. In G. V. Coelho, D. A. Hamburg, & J. E. Adams (Eds.), *Coping and adaptation* (pp. 249–315). New York: Basic Books.

Lazarus, R. S., & Launier, R. (1978). Stress-related transactions between person and environment. In L. A. Pervin & M. Lewis (Eds.), *Perspectives in interactional psychology* (pp. 287–327). New York: Plenum Press.
Levine, S. (1985). A definition of stress? In G. P. Moberg (Ed.), *Animal stress* (pp. 51–69) Bethesda, MD: American Physiological Society.
Levine, S. (1987). Psychobiologic consequences of mother–infant relationships. In N. Krasnegor, E. Blass, M. Hofer, & W. Smotherman (Eds.), *Perinatal development: A psychobiological perspective* (pp. 359–376). New York: Academic Press.
Levine, S., Coe, C. L., Smotherman, W. P., & Kaplan, J. N. (1978). Prolonged cortisol elevation in the infant squirrel monkey after reunion with mother. *Physiology & Behavior, 20,* 7–10.
Levine, S., Franklin, D., & Gonzales, C. A. (1984). Influence of social variables on the biobehavioral response to separation in rhesus monkey infants. *Child Development, 55,* 1386–1393.
Levine, S., Goldman, L., & Coover, G. D. (1972). Expectancy and the pituitary–adrenal system. In R. Porter & J. Knight (Eds.), *Physiology, emotion and psychosomatic illness* (Ciba Foundation Symposium) (pp. 281–296). Amsterdam: Elsevier.
Levine, S., Johnson, D. F., & Gonzales, C. A. (1985). Behavioral and hormonal responses to separation in infant rhesus monkeys and mothers. *Behavioral Neuroscience, 99,* 399–410.
Levine, S., & Wiener, S. G. (1988). Psychoendocrine aspects of mother–infant relationships in nonhuman primates. *Psychoneuroendocrinology, 13*: 143–154.
Lewis, M., & Goldberg, S. (1969). Perceptual-cognitive development in infancy: A generalized expectancy model as a function of the mother-infant interaction. *Merrill–Palmer Quarterly, 15,* 81–100.
Mason, W. A. (1978). Social experience in primate cognitive development. In G. M. Burghardt & M. Bekoff (Eds.), *The development of behavior: Comparative and evolutionary aspects* (pp. 233–251). New York: Garland STPM Press.
McGinnis, L. M. (1980). Maternal separation studies in children and nonhuman primates. In R. W. Bell & W. P. Smotherman (Eds.), *Maternal influences and early behavior* (pp. 311–336). New York: Spectrum.
Mendoza, S. P., Smotherman, W. P., Miner, M. T., Kaplan, J. N., & Levine, S. (1978). Pituitary–adrenal response to separation in mother and infant squirrel monkeys. *Developmental Psychobiology, 11,* 169–175.
Mineka, S., & Suomi, S. J. (1978). Social separation in monkeys. *Psychological Bulletin, 85,* 1376–1400.
Munck, A., Guyre, P. M., & Holbrook, N. J. (1984). Physiological functions of glucocorticoids in stress and their relation to pharmacological actions. *Endocrine Reviews, 5,* 25–44.
Pribram, K. H., & Melges, F. T. (1969). Psychophysiological basis of emotion. In P. J. Vinken & G. W. Bruyn (Eds.), *Handbook of clinical neurology* (pp. 316–342). Amsterdam: North-Holland.
Reite, M., Short, R., & Seiler, C. (1978). Physiological correlates of maternal separation in surrogate-reared infants: A study in altered attachment bonds. *Developmental Psychobiology, 11,* 427–435.

Roberston, J., & Robertson, J. (1971). Young children in brief separation: A fresh look. *Psychoanalytic Study of the Child, 26*, 264–315.

Rosenblum, L. A., Plimpton, E. H. (1981). Adaptation to separation: The infant's effort to cope with an altered environment. In M. Lewis & L. A. Rosenblum (Eds.), *The uncommon child: Genesis of behavior* (pp. 225–257). New York: Plenum Press.

Seay, B. M., & Harlow, H. F. (1965). Maternal separation in the rhesus monkey. *Journal of Nervous and Mental Diseases, 140*, 434–441.

Sokolov, E. N. (1960). Neuronal models and the orienting reflex. In M. A. B. Brazier (Ed.), *The central nervous system and behavior.* (pp. 187–276). New York: Josiah Macy, Jr. Foundation.

Stanton, M. E., Patterson, J. M., & Levine, S. (1985). Social influences on conditioned cortisol secretion in the squirrel monkey. *Psychoneuroendocrinology, 10*, 125–134.

Suomi, S. J., Collins, M. L., Harlow, H. F., & Ruppenthal, G. C. (1976). Effects of maternal and peer separations on young monkeys. *Journal of Child Psychology and Psychiatry, 17*, 101–112.

Weinberg, J., & Levine, S. (1980). Psychobiology of coping in animals: The effects of predictability. In S. Levine & H. Ursin (Eds.), *Coping and health* (pp. 39–59). New York: Plenum Press.

Weinraub, M., & Lewis, M. (1977). The determinants of children's responses to separation. *Monographs in Social Research on Child Development, 42*, 172.

Weiss, J. M. (1971a). Effects of coping behavior in different warning signal conditions on stress pathology in rats. *Journal of Comparative and Physiological Psychology, 77*, 1–13.

Weiss, J. M. (1971b). Effects of punishing the coping response (conflict) on stress pathology in rats. *Journal of Comparative and Physiological Psychology, 77*, 14–21.

Weiss, J. M. (1971c). Effects of coping behavior with and without a feedback signal on stress pathology in rats. *Journal of Comparative and Physiological Psychology, 77*, 22–30.

Weiss, J. M. (1972). Influence of psychological variables on stress-induced pathology. In R. Porter & J. Knight (Eds.), *Physiology, emotion & pyschosomatic illness* (pp. 253–279; 393–394). Amsterdam: Elsevier.

Wiener, S. G., Johnson, D. F., & Levine, S. (1987). Influence of postnatal rearing conditions on the response of squirrel monkey infants to brief perturbations in mother-infant relationships. *Physiological Behavior, 39*, 21–26.

2

The Physiology of Stress and Behavioral Development

Elizabeth J. Susman
The Pennsylvania State University

Editha D. Nottelmann
National Institute of Mental Health

Lorah D. Dorn
The Pennsylvania State University

Philip W. Gold
National Institute of Mental Health

George P. Chrousos
National Institute of Child Health and Human Development

Stress (a state of threatened homeostasis) has been implicated in the onset of physical illness and psychiatric disorders in individuals of all age groups. Recent research in several disciplines, including developmental psychology, endocrinology, and psychiatry, has begun to examine the processes linking environmental stressors (threats against homeostasis), the physiology of the stress response and physical illness, psychiatric disorders, and behavioral development in general. In this chapter, we examine first the physiological responses to stress as a mechanism whereby environmental stressors may affect the course of behavioral development throughout the life span. Next, we discuss individual differences in reactivity to stressors. The physiological processes involved in our formulations of stress reactivity are primarily those involving the interactions between hormones of adrenal and gonadal origin. Finally, we examine stressors in three domains in which stress-related physiological changes may lead to alterations in behavioral development: (a) social and emotional stressors during adolescence; (b) physical stressors, with exercise as a paradigm; and (c) stressors associated with affective disorders. As the literature in these three areas is too extensive for a review here, we use examples from our own research and from the research of colleagues to illustrate potential links between the physiology of stress and behavioral development.

In examining issues involved in interrelations of the physiology of stress and behavioral development, we assume the following: (a) There is great individual variability in both physiological and behavioral reactions to comparable stressors. These individual differences may determine whether stressors will influence the course of behavioral development. (b) The physiological aspects of the stress response may affect behavioral development directly (e.g., by producing pathophysiological changes in organs and tissues) and indirectly, by altering psychological development as a result of stress-related changes in physiological systems (e.g., by altering the timing of some aspect of a normal developmental sequence).

PHYSIOLOGY OF THE STRESS RESPONSE

In response to stressors, and with the ultimate goal of adapting to new situations and attaining homeostasis, the mammalian organism has to alter its behavior as well as its physiologic state. Behavioral changes include heightened activity, increased vigilance, and decreased feeding and reproductive behavior. On a teleological basis, these changes may enhance the chance of survival. Similar teleology can be ascribed to physiological changes. The central nervous system (CNS) is the coordination center that senses stressors and orchestrates the stress response. Physiological changes include the improvement of nutrition, and oxygenation and detoxification of the CNS and any other organ involved in the fight or flight response, for instance, a specific group of muscles that is activated during the stress of strenuous exercise.

Major centers in the CNS that appear to be effectors for both the behavioral and the physiological component of the stress response include the hypothalamic corticotropin releasing hormone (CRH) neurons (primarily paraventricular nucleus), the hypothalamic proopiomelanocortin (POMC) neurons in the arcuate nucleus, and the central sympathetic nuclei of the hindbrain (locus coeruleus [LC] and others). (See Fig. 2.1.) The CRH neuron is responsible for stimulating the pituitary corticotroph to secrete adrenocorticotropin hormone (ACTH) and consequently the adrenal cortex to secrete cortisol and androgens. The same neuron also activates the hypothalamic POMC neuron to secrete ACTH and β-endorphin and the locus coeruleus and other sympathetic nuclei to secrete catecholamines. Locus coeruleus activation by CRH causes not only arousal, but also activation of the CRH neuron itself (Britton, Koob, Rivier, & Vale, 1982; Calogero, Gallucci, Gold, & Chrousos, 1988a, 1988b; Sutton, Koob, LeMoal, Rivier, & Vale, 1982; Valentino, Foote, & Aston-Jones, 1983). Central sympathetic system activation by CRH also causes peripheral catecholamine secretion (Brown et al., 1982). Catecholamines are the principle modulators of cardiovascular function, as well as the major mediators of the fight or flight response.

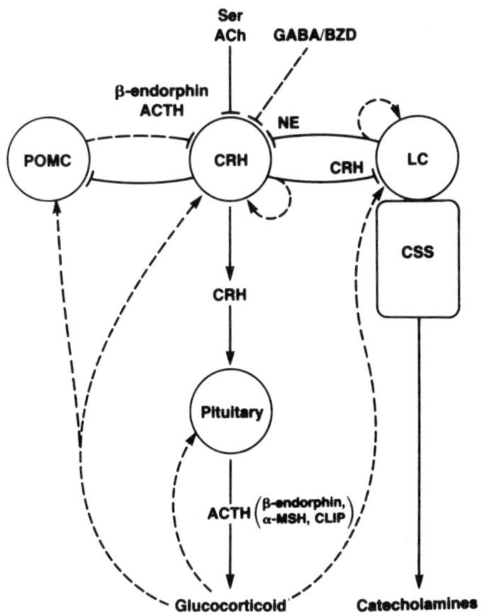

FIG. 2.1. A schematic representation of the two major neuroendocrine systems involved in the stress response. The major modifier of hypothalamic-pituitary-adrenocortical activity appears to be the hypothalamic neurons responsible for secretion of CRH. This neuropeptide is involved not only in the stimulation of pituitary adrenocorticotropic hormone (ACTH) secretion but also in the activation of the locus coeruleus (LC) and other sympathetic system (CSS) nuclei in the brain stem. Activation of these centers leads to increased arousal and increased catecholamine secretion in the periphery by the adrenal medulla and the sympathetic nerve terminals. Moreover, CRH stimulates the proopiomelanocortin neurons in the hypothalamic arcuate nucleus leading to increased secretion of ACTH and β-endorphin. The major stimulants of hypothalamic CRH secretion are norepinephrine (NE), serotonin (Ser), and acetylcholine (Ach). Inhibitors of CRH secretion include CRH, GABA, opioid peptides, ACTH and cortisol. Cortisol is also involved in feedback inhibition of the POMC neuron, the pituitary corticotroph and the LC. Uninterrupted lines indicate stimulation, interrupted lines indicate inhibition. Arrowheads indicate endocrine effect, tau shaped lines indicate neuronal effect.

A large number of interactions between the various mediators of the stress response is shown in Fig. 2.1. Glucocorticoid hormones play a major negative feedback role, possibly participating in the restraint of the stress response. Another restraining role of glucocorticoids during the stress response is that exerted by these hormones on the immune system. Munck, Guyre, and Holbrook (1984) have suggested that glucocorticoids are elevated during immune–inflammatory responses in order to protect the organism from excessive reactions.

Although the schematic representation of the various interrelations of the various effectors and mediators of the stress response in Fig. 2.1 is supported by many studies, its primary value is heuristic. The figure shows that the stress system is interrelated with components of the reproductive axis. As discussed later, it appears that one of the mechanisms by which stress influences reproductive function is via CRH-stimulated secretion of POMC neuron β-endorphin, which causes suppression of the hypothalamic luteinizing hormone releasing hormone neuron.

INDIVIDUAL DIFFERENCES IN STRESS REACTIVITY

Although all individuals confront a variety of comparable stressors throughout their life span, some individuals cope with these stressors with a minimum of physiological or psychological sequelae, whereas others develop physical or psychiatric illness. In considering individual differences in stress reactivity, responses to normative stressors (daily hassles) as well as to major stressors are included as potential influences on behavioral development. Normative minor stressors that are enduring may have as deleterious an effect on development as the major stressors examined in much of the previous literature (e.g., soldiers in battle). That is, we propose that the processes linking the physiology of stress and behavioral development may be similar regardless of the magnitude of the stressor.

One-major focus of the stress and coping literature has been on individual differences in reactivity to environmental stressors under conditions involving uncertainty or novel and challenging conditions. Exaggerated or heightened physiological and behavioral reactivity to novel and challenging stimuli, that is not evident in familiar and/or normative environmental settings (Suomi, 1987), is characteristic of some animals and humans. Exaggerated or heightened reactivity is considered a vulnerability factor in development (e.g., Levine, 1984). The explanations for exaggerated reactivity include genetic factors (Plomin & Stocker, in press), temperament (Thomas, Chess, & Korn, 1982), and low threshold of responsitivity in limbic and hypothalamic structures (Kagan, Resnick, & Snidman, 1987). Although there is no consensus regarding the basis for individual differences in reactivity, there is general agreement that heightened reactivity may be important for three reasons. Heightened physiological and behavioral reactivity may be involved in, and serve as, a marker for identifying individuals at risk for the development of anxiety, depression, or other affective disorders (Suomi 1987). Heightened reactivity also may be involved in the development of physical disease (e.g., cardiovascular disease) (Williams, 1986). In addition, heightened reactivity may reflect and also influence psychosocial adjustment and interpersonal relations, (i.e., relationships with peers) (Kagan et al., 1987) and relationships in the family. Thus, individual differences in physiological and behavioral reactivity to environmental stressors have important implications for the larger question of whether and how physiological or behavioral reactivity to novel and challenging conditions is related to social and emotional development in general and to the development of psychiatric disorders in particular.

Among the many studies that have examined individual differences in reactivity to novel and challenging situations, one series of studies with primates elegantly demonstrates the physiological and behavioral manifestations of exaggerated reactivity (Suomi, 1984, 1987). This series of studies shows that some monkeys characteristically show heightened physiological and behavioral responses when confronted with novel and challenging (stressor) situations. The physiological reactions of these monkeys include extreme and prolonged elevations in plasma ACTH and cortisol, and elevated and stable heart rates following separation from their attachment objects. Their behavioral reactions include low levels of locomotion, exploration, play, and vocalization. This pattern of reactivity characteristics was found to be stable from infancy to adolescence and was related to anxiety and/or depression-like behaviors. However, the parameters that distinguished these highly reactive from less reactive monkeys were present only during times of environmental challenge (Suomi, 1987).

The explanations for exaggerated reactivity in rhesus monkeys, as in humans, include genetic and environmental components. The latter includes, for example, the physiological reactivity characteristics of the mother as well as mothering style (e.g., nurturant versus punitive behavior). Suomi and colleagues (1987) examined the genetic and environmental bases for differences in behavioral and physiological responses to challenge in a cross-fostering study. Infants were selected for the study on the basis of their genetic pedigree. Half of the infants had biological parents who had consistently produced highly reactive offspring. The other half had biological parents who consistently produced moderately reactive offspring. Both sets of infants were separated from their biological mothers at birth to be reared by foster mothers.

The infants of highly reactive biological parents achieved lower orienting scores, had somewhat poorer muscle tonus and were less advanced in motor reflexes, and displayed greater inhibition than the infants of less reactive biological parents. At 6 months, when the infants were separated from their foster mothers, infants of parents who had produced highly reactive offspring responded to the separation with heightened behavioral (longer periods of passivity) and physiological reactivity (higher levels of cortisol) reactivity compared to infants of parents who had produced less reactive offspring. Differences in the maternal style of the foster mother were not reflected in the infant responses. In brief, the genetic pedigree of the infants was a better predictor of individual differences in their reactivity than reactivity characteristics and/or the mothering style of the foster mothers.

The transmission of individual differences in reactivity characteristics in humans is less well understood. In the absence of research designed to examine genetic and environmental factors in reactivity, theoretical notions about their respective or cumulative roles in individual differences in reactivity remain as speculation. Nonetheless, the high incidence of intergenerational transmission of physical health and psychiatric disorders (e.g., depression) suggests that perhaps reactivity tendencies, comparable to the exaggerated, apparently heritable reactivity characteristics in the anxiety or depression prone rhesus monkeys, may be heritable also in humans as in subhuman primates.

STRESS AND GONADAL FUNCTIONING: IMPLICATIONS FOR PHYSICAL DEVELOPMENT

The interaction of the hypothalamic-pituitary-adrenal axis (HPA), the physiological system activated by environmental stressors, and the hypothalamic-pituitary-gonadal axis (HPG), the physiological system responsible for reproductive functioning, has special relevance for the timely progression of behavioral development. The exceedingly complex interaction between the HPA and HPG axes is regulated by positive and negative influence systems involving the hypothalamus, pituitary, adrenal glands, and gonads. In both animals and humans, activation of the HPA axis is associated with suppression of the HPG axis. Figure 2.2 shows the possible linkages between environmental stressors, the HPA axis, the HPG axis, and physical maturation and reproductive function. HPA activation and associated alterations in gonadal functioning may have implications for fetal development; the timing and progression of physical growth, especially at puberty; the timing of menarche and regularity of menstrual cycles; and cognitive, social, and emotional development. Thus, the physiological aspects of stress as mediated by gonadal functioning may influence the course of behavioral development in ways that have not been considered previously.

The pioneering work of Cannon (1929), Selye (1950), and others clearly established that both physical and psychological factors resulted in adrenal activation. The influence of stress on gonadal activation was later to be described during fetal, pubertal, and adult life. In animal studies (see Collu, Gibb, & Ducharme, 1984, for a review), exposure of animals to physical stressors or peripheral administration of corticotropin releasing factor (CRF) have been used to demonstrate the effects of stress on gonadal functioning. Specifically, in rats, immobilization or handling stress has been shown to induce a fall in plasma concentration of testosterone (T) (Charpenet et al., 1981) and

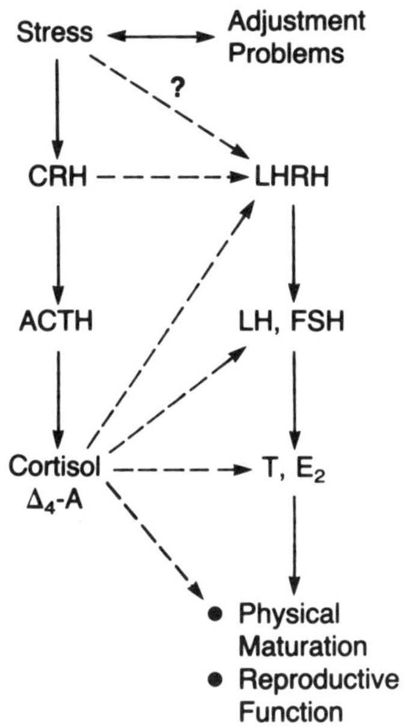

FIG. 2.2. A schematic representation of the two neuroendocrine axes that are implicated in behavior changes during adolescence. The hypothalamic-pituitary-adrenal axis (left) is activated during physical or emotional stress. It is responsible for the secretion of hypothalamic corticotropin releasing hormone (CRH), pituitary adrenocorticotropin hormone (ACTH) and adrenal cortisol and adrenal androgens, such as androstenedione (△4–A).

The hypothalamic-pituitary-gonadal axis (HPG) (right), is responsible for the secretion of luteinizing hormone (LH) and follicle stimulating hormone (FSH), and the gonadal steroids, testosterone (T), estradiol (E_2), and progesterone. The HPG is responsible for the physical maturation at puberty and maintenance of reproductive function.

The solid lines indicate stimulation. The interrupted lines indicate suppression. (From Nottelmann, Inoff-Germain, Susman, & Chrousos, in press.)

altered testicular steroidogenesis during puberty (Collu et al., 1984). The effects of handling and other stressors (e.g., injections of saline) affected not only gonadal steroid secretion but also secretion of gonadotropins, growth hormone, and prolactin (Krulich, Hefco, Illner, & Read, 1974). Furthermore, acute infusion of CRF into female rats caused inhibition of (LH) lutenizing hormone (but not follicle stimulating hormone–FSH), inhibition of ovulation, and disruption of pregnancy (Rivier & Vale, 1984). Long-term administration of CRF to male rats caused inhibition of LH, T, and prolactin secretion, and decreased seminal vesicle weights (Rivier & Vale, 1985). Similarly, in ovariectomized rhesus monkeys, administration of CRH led to decreased levels of LH and FSH secretion, an effect that can be blocked by opioid antagonists. These findings support the hypothesis that elevated CRH levels may contribute to alterations in reproductive functioning (Olster & Ferin, 1987).

Similarly, in adult humans, activation of the HPA axis is related to suppression of the HPG axis as well. Higher levels of cortisol have been found to be related to lower levels of LH in males and females (Sakakura, Takebe, & Nakagawa, 1975; Sowers, Rice, & Blanchard, 1979) and lower levels of T in males (Cumming, Quigley, & Yen, 1983; Francis, 1981; Schaison, Durand, & Mowszowicz, 1978). In addition, lower levels of T were found in males with higher (vs. lower) self-reported levels of stress than in males with lower levels of stress (Francis, 1981). This latter finding is unique in that there are few empirical findings linking the emotional, subjective, and biological aspects of stress.

The evolutionary value of the pattern of activation of the HPA axis and suppression of the HPG axis at first seems antithetical to species survival. Long-term activation of the HPA axis at the expense of suppression of the HPG axis could prevent species reproduction. However, short-term adrenocortical activation as part of the defense reaction or fight and flight mechanism is consistent with survival and in order to mobilize resources for the defense reaction, reproductive functions become compromised, at least in the short term.

Social and Emotional Stressors. Adolescence has been identified as an inhererently stressful period of development (Hamburg, 1974). New challenges converge during the adolescent years that may become multiple new stressors. These challenges include new demands in school, changing peer-group dynamics, and adjustment in family relationships (Brooks-Gunn, 1987; Petersen, 1987). That adolescence is stressful is supported by an increase in psychiatric disorders during that period of development (Carlson & Cantwell, 1978; Rutter, Graham, Chadwick, & Yule, 1976). Puberty itself, occurring between ages 9 and 15, is considered to be a source of stress because of the associated changes in hormone levels, height, weight, and body contour. Increases in the levels of puberty-related hormones, for instance, are assumed to have both direct and indirect effects on behavior (Petersen & Taylor, 1980). The direct effects hypothesis suggests that increases in the levels of gonadal and adrenal axis hormones may influence behavior through alterations in neurotransmitters, neurotransmitter receptor sites, or other unknown biological processes in the brain. The indirect effects hypothesis suggests that behavior changes are mediated through changes in physical growth and related social processes. That is, external manifestations of puberty signal to parents, peers, and others that the adolescent has a new status, one which they expect to be accompanied by more independent and responsible behavior. Such expectations, in turn, are likely to influence the adolescent's behavior.

Few studies have concentrated on the influence of hormones as contributors to the stressfulness of adolescence. Until recently, hypotheses about hormone and behavior links have focused on hormones of gonadal origin in male participants (e.g., Olweus, 1986). A broader array of hormones in females and males currently are being examined (Brooks–Gunn & Warren, in press; Nottelmann et al., 1987; Susman et al., 1985). In our own study of hormone changes and psychological development in young adolescents, we hypothesized that hormones of adrenal origin, as well as hormones of gonadal origin, were important to consider as possible influences on the behavioral changes that occur in young adolescents. Although androgens of adrenal origin generally are considered to be biologically weak androgens, it seems important to consider their relation to psychological development during adolescence because adrenal androgen secretion may reflect environmental stressor-related activation of the HPA.

A pattern of findings emerged in our study that appears to link the stressors of pubertal development and adrenal and gonadal hormones. We examined the interrelations among hormones of gonadal and adrenal origin, physical maturation, and social and emotional development in young adolescents. The sample consisted of 108 healthy adolescents: 56 boys, ages 10–14 years, and 52 girls, ages 9–14 years. There were three assessments, at 6-month intervals of physical maturity, endocrine status, and psychological and behavioral functioning. The adolescents were assessed on psychological dimensions hypothesized to be related to hormone changes at adolescence, including aggression, self-image, moods, cognition, behavior problems, and qualitative aspects of parent-adolescent interactions. The adolescents had a physical examination to assess their stage of pubertal development (Tanner criteria, Marshall & Tanner, 1969, 1970), as well as height, weight, and head circumference for both genders, and testicular volume (Prader orchidometer) for boys. For the hormone level assessment, blood samples were collected between the hours of 8 and 10 a.m. to minimize the effects of diurnal variations on the levels of the hormones that were measured. For each adolescent, a sample was drawn at 0, 20, and 40 minutes.

In one aspect of the study, the relations between adrenal and gonadal axis hormones, emotional dispositions, and aggressive attributes were examined (Susman et al., 1987). The hypothesis tested was that higher levels of androgens (primarily T, and to a lesser extent the adrenal androgens) are related to higher levels of aggressive behavior. Negative emotions were assumed to be involved in the pathway between hormone levels and aggressive behavior. The general pattern of findings was that, for boys only, a profile of lower gonadal steroid levels and higher androstenedione (△4–A) levels was related to acting out and aggressive behavior. For instance, lower estradiol (E_2)levels, a lower testosterone to estradiol ratio (T/E_2), lower testosterone–estradiol binding globulin (TeBG), and higher levels of △4–A were associated with more acting out behavior problems. Anxiety was the emotion related to acting out behavior problems. There were no associations in girls among hormones, emotions, and aggressive behavior.

Similarly, from the same sample of young adolescents, Nottelmann and colleagues (Nottelmann et al., 1987), reported that adjustment problems were associated with a hormone profile of higher △4–A levels and either lower T levels or a lower T/E_2 ratio. When age and/or pubertal stage were controlled, the associations between hormone levels and adjustment problems remained relatively constant. The hormone and chronological age profile associated with adjustment problems was characteristic of later maturation, relatively lower sex steroid levels, or lower pubertal stage, and relatively higher △4–A levels, sometimes in conjunction with higher chronological age. Thus, adjustment problems were more likely in males with later maturation, lower gonadal steroid levels for chronological age, and lower pubertal stage for chronological age.

A profile of lower gonadal steroid levels and negative emotions and adjustment and behavior problems, in conjunction with lower pubertal stage, is consistent with the literature linking stress and gonadal functioning in both animals and humans. Although the types of stressors encountered in healthy adolescents might be considered minor compared to the types of stressors considered in past studies on the physiology of stress and behavior, minor stressors (daily hassles that elicit strong emotions in adolescents) may be sufficient to alter slightly the course of pubertal development. Thus, it is not beyond reason that the stress experienced by some adolescents affects their tempo of pubertal development (Nottelmann, Inoff-Germain, Susman, & Chrousos, in press; Susman, Nottelmann, Inoff-Germain, Dorn, & Chrousos, in press). Potential stressor-related alterations in the changes in hormone levels during puberty are reflected in Fig. 2.3. The solid lines represent the normal developmental trajectory of the hormones. The broken lines represent the atypical developmental trajectory of the hormones under conditions of chronic stress. Alternatively, later maturation may be a chronic stressor in young adolescents, particularly males. Associations have been reported for adolescents between relatively poor self-perceptions that may reflect adjustment problems and lagging pubertal development and physical growth. Blyth and colleagues (Blyth et al., 1981) reported that later pubertal development in males is related to lower levels of body image and self-esteem for boys. Similarly, Nottelmann (1982) found that males who were less mature than most of their age mates (based on a weight and height index of physical maturity) saw themselves as being relatively low in academic competence.

The relatively minor chronic stressors encountered by adolescents may be reflected in the higher levels of △4–A that we observed in the later maturing boys. Androstenedione is closely linked to cortisol production under conditions of chronic stress. Fig. 2.4 shows a schematic representation between CRH, ACTH, △4–A, and the putative adrenal androgen stimulating factor and the other adrenal androgens of the △5 series, including dehydroepiandrosterone (DHEA) and dehydroepiandrosterone sulphate (DHEAS). The bold arrows

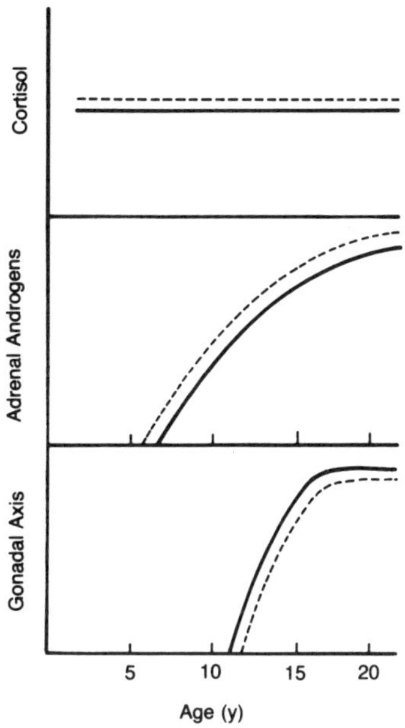

FIG. 2.3. A schematic representation of the relative activity of the hypothalamic-pituitary-adrenal and hypothalamic-pituitary-gonadal axes under conditions of higher and lower levels of stress. Cortisol secretion remains relatively constant during childhood and adolescence (top panel). Adrenal androgen secretion starts at approximately 6 years and reaches peak levels at approximately 20 years of age (middle panel). Gonadal steroid secretion starts at 11 years and reaches peak levels at 16 years of age (bottom panel). The solid lines represent individuals with lower levels of stress. The interrupted lines represent individuals with higher levels of chronic stress. (From Nottelmann, Inoff-Germain, Susman, & Chrousos, in press.)

indicate that ACTH has a much more potent influence on △4–A than on DHEA or DHEAS. Thus, it seems reasonable that the relations between adjustment problems and △4–A should be more pronounced than those between adjustment problems and DHEA or DHEAS (Nottelmann et al., in press).

Although the secretion of △4–A and cortisol secretion both are linked to adrenal activation, much less is known about △4–A and behavior than about cortisol and behavior. A large body of literature in man and animals shows links between adrenal activation, as reflected in cortisol levels, and distress behavior (e.g., Mason, 1968; Rose, 1980; Suomi, 1987). Briefly, the links between adrenal activation and cortisol production generally occur in novel and challenging situations and disappear when the situation becomes familiar (e.g., Levine, 1984; Mason, 1968). We are beginning to examine in detail the

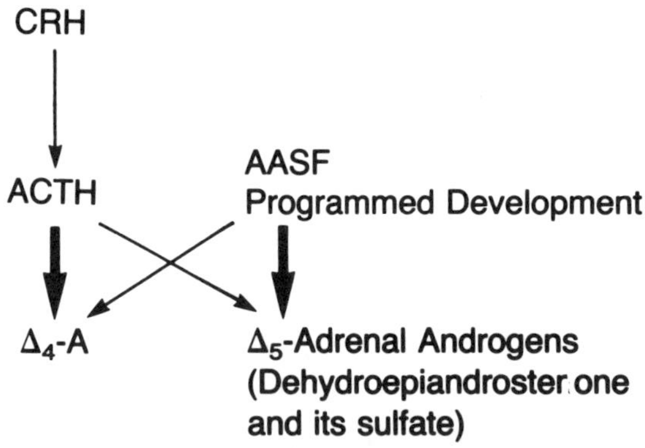

FIG. 2.4. A schematic representation of adrenal androgen regulation. A putative hormone, adrenal androgen stimulating factor (AASF), has been proposed as regulator of *zona reticularis* growth and function. Development of this zone occurs between 4 to 5 and 20 years of age. Alternatively, genetically programmed development of *zona reticularis* cells may explain its age related growth. All adrenal androgens (androstenedione and dehydroepiandrosterone or dehydroepiandrosterone sulphate) are dependent on ACTH stimulation of the adrenal *zona reticularis*. It appears that △4–A is more ACTH dependent than are the △5–adrenal androgens (bold arrow). This link is supported by the finding that △4-steroids like cortisol and △4–A are elevated at the expense of decreased secretion of △5 adrenal androgens (Parker, Levin, & Lifrak, 1985). (From Nottelmann, Inoff-Germain, Susman, & Chrousos, in press.)

consistency in relations between cortisol levels and △4–A. These relations are being examined from the same three samples of blood, obtained at each of the three times of assessment, at 6-month intervals. For boys, △4–A and cortisol levels were significantly correlated ($p \leq .05$) at time one of assessment in sample one, two, and three; at time two of assessment, there were no significant correlations between △4–A and cortisol; at time three of assessment, △4–A and cortisol levels were significantly correlated in samples one and three. For girls, there were no relations between cortisol and △4–A levels in any of the samples at any of the three times of assessment. The lack of associations in girls may reflect the fact that a significant proportion of △4–A is secreted by the ovaries whose function might, in fact, be affected negatively by a hyperactive HPA axis.

In summary, the potential role of △4–A as part of the stress response and its relation to behavior is just beginning to be examined. However, the consistency of our findings relating △4–A levels to poor adjustment in male adolescents, and very recent research findings in animals, suggest that the study of its efficacy and functional significance in influencing behavior might be an intereresting research avenue. Currently, Glickman, Frank, Davidson, Smith, and Siiteri (1987) are examining relations between circulating levels of △4–A and behavior relations in a colony of spotted hyenas. Female spotted hyenas are characterized by high levels of △4–A and high levels of aggression. The study of the developmental changes in △4–A and aggressiveness in the spotted hyenas may lead to new models for examining the △4–A behavior link in humans.

Physical Exercise Stress. Physical exercise, such as intensive running and dancing, activates the HPA axis and presents a challenge to homeostasis (Luger et al., 1987). Physical stress resulting from rigorous exercise may affect physiological mechanisms that may, in turn, alter the course of behavioral development.

In runners, the degree of acute HPA activation in response to stress is inversely proportional to the degree of physical fitness of the individual (Luger et al., 1987). However, compared to moderately trained runners and sedentary individuals, obligate runners who run over 45 miles per week have elevated evening concentrations of plasma ACTH and cortisol. They also have elevated values of 24 hour urinary cortisol excretion. Figure 2.5 shows mean ACTH, cortisol, and lactate in untrained, moderately trained, and highly trained runners.

The link between HPA activation and gonadal functioning has been established in exercise. An earlier study of runners showed clear links between running a marathon and adrenocortical and gonadal functioning (Dessypris, Kuoppasalmi, & Adlercreutz, 1976). After the run, there were significant mean increases in cortisol and △4–A and significant decreases in T. Luteinizing hormone was decreased after the marathon. One of the conclusions was that androgens and cortisol act to promote endurance in men.

The recently described hypercortisolism in highly trained runners is of similar magnitude to the hypercortisolism observed in anorexia nervosa or depression (Gold, Gwirtsman et al., 1986; Gold, Loriaux et al., 1986). Thus, running, per se, may not be the cause of elevated levels of ACTH and cortisol (Luger et al., 1987) but rather a method of coping with anorectic or depressive tendencies. Interestingly, highly trained runners have some degree of hypothalamic hypogonadism (MacConnie, Barkan, Lampman, Schork, & Beitins, 1986) similar to that observed in anorexia nervosa.

In highly dedicated dancers, the physical stress undoubtedly is related systematically to activation of the HPA axis through mechanisms similar to those in runners. The effects of the physical stress of the demanding exercise regimen of dancers on growth and development appear to be mediated through gonadal functioning (Brooks-Gunn & Warren, 1985; Brooks-Gunn, 1987; Warren, 1980; Warren, Brooks-Gunn, Hamilton, Hamilton, & Warren, 1986). Specifically, pubertal progression, including menarche, appears to be influenced by the rigors of ballet dancing (Warren, 1980). In the Brooks-Gunn and Warren program of research, more dance students than nondance students were late maturers, and the dancers weighed less and were leaner than the nondance students (Brooks-Gunn & Warren, 1985). Furthermore, the behavior of the dancers was characterized by less favorable family relationships and more difficulties with impulse control (Brooks-Gunn, 1987). The dancers also were

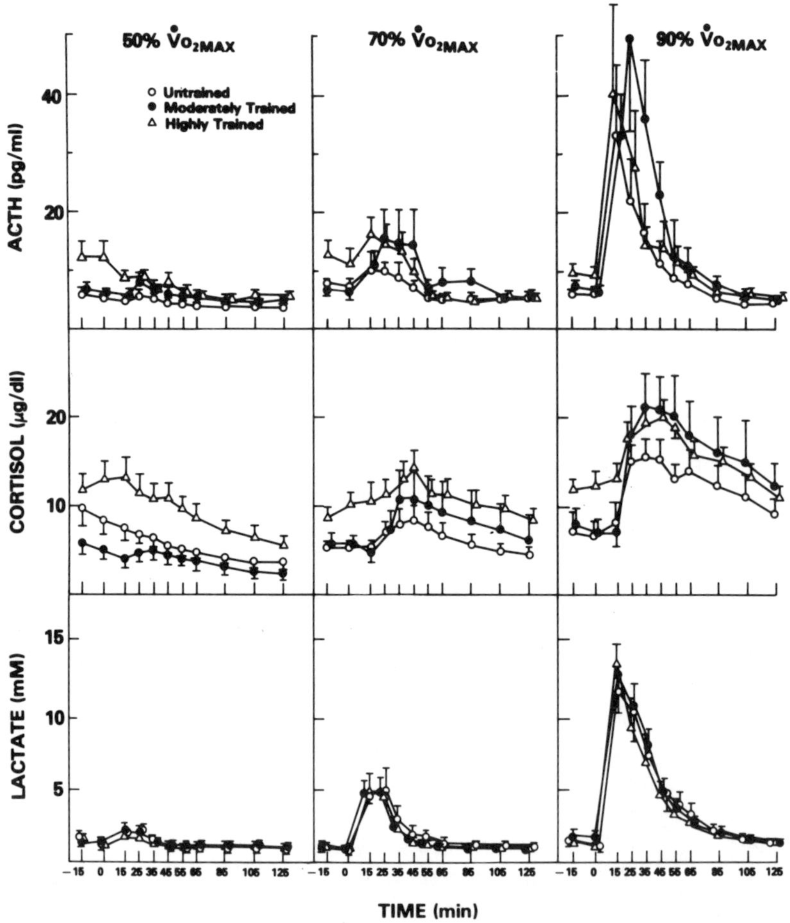

FIG. 2.5 Mean ± plasma ACTH (top panels), cortisol (middle panels) and lactate (bottom panels) in three groups of subjects (untrained and moderately and highly trained male runners) receiving treadmill exercise at 50% ∇O_2 max, 70% ∇O_2 max, and 90% ∇O2 max. Basal plasma ACTH and cortisol were elevated in the highly trained runners. The same individuals had elevated 24-hour urinary free cortisol excretion and blunted ACTH and cortisol responses to oCRH, findings suggesting mildly hypercortisolism in highly trained athletes. (From Luger et al., 1987). Reprinted with permission of *The New England Journal of Medicine.*

less likely to date than other same-age students. Whereas menarche had no effect on dating behavior in nondancers, postmenarcheal dancers were more likely to date than premenarcheal dancers.

These and other findings from the same program of research, suggest the complex interactions between a particular physical stressor, in this case dancing, and the physiological sequelae of that stressor and behavioral development. What is unclear is the direction of causal influences among delayed biological-pubertal processes, dancing, and behavioral development. Although one might be tempted to conclude that physical stress suppresses gonadal functioning and related pubertal processes, girls may continue with ballet because they are late maturers which accords them certain weight and height advantages over early maturers.

STRESS AND PSYCHIATRIC DISORDERS

The question of whether environmental stressors and psychiatric disorders, particularly affective disorders, occur in antecedent-consequent relations has existed for decades. Anisman and Lapierre (1982) reviewed the basic positions they and others developed over the years relating stress and affective disorders: (a) stress is not a precipitating factor in clinical depression; (b) depressed individuals possess a heightened reactivity to stressors; (c) stress may provoke depression, given that individuals have a genetic predisposition; (d) stress may induce depression if the ability to cope with stressors has not been developed; and; (e) stress does not influence the variety of types of depression in the same way, as stress does not affect all individuals in the same way.

Recent studies of the neuroendocrinology of psychiatric disorders suggest links between the physiology of the stress response and the pathophysiology of psychiatric disorders. Hypercortisolism, a characteristic response to environmental stressors, also is associated with psychiatric disorders, namely depression and anorexia nervosa (Chrousos et al., 1987; Gold & Chrousos, 1985; Gold, Goodwin, & Chrousos, in press; Gold, Gwirtsman et al., 1986; Gold, Loriaux et al., 1986). Depressed patients showed elevated cortisol levels and a blunted response to ovine CRH. Underweight patients with anorexia nervosa showed even more severe hypercortisolism than that observed in depressed patients, (Gold, Loriaux et al., 1986). Anorectics also showed marked attenuation of the plasma ACTH response to exogenous CRH. The interpretation of the finding in which hypercortisolism was associated with an attenuated response to CRH in depressed as well as anorexic individuals is that there is hypersecretion in these patients. The CRH hypersecretion leads to hypercortisolism and restrained pituitary corticotroph cell response to exogenous CRH as a result of increased negative feedback exerted by the elevated cortisol levels (Gold, Gwirtsman et al., 1986; Gold, Loriaux et al., 1986).

Although empirically derived relations between hypercortisolism in response to stressors in general and affective disorders in particular have not been firmly established, evidence from several disciplines suggests these links. First, laboratory animals exposed to maternal deprivation early in life show hyperactivity of the HPA axis later in life (e.g., Thomas, Levine, & Arnold, 1968). Second, in humans, depression-prone individuals are likely to report greater than average early traumatic experiences or maternal deprivation. In squirrel monkeys, maternal deprivation evokes pituitary-adrenal activation equal to or greater than that induced by physical trauma (Coe, Wiener, Rosenberg, & Levine, 1985). In this species of monkeys, there was marked adrenal activation following 30-minute separations from mother (Levine, Coe, Smotherman, & Kaplan, 1978). Cortisol elevations following separation lasted for six hours, even when behavioral agitation decreased (Coe, Wiener, & Levine, 1983). These early stressors may sensitize or entrain the adrenal axis to hyperreact to environmental stressors leading to hypersecretion of cortisol in the presence of similar stressors throughout the lifespan. Third, there is the notion that there are kindling changes in susceptibility to stress (Gold, Goodwin, & Chrousos, in press). That is, given temperamental or genetic predispositions, sensitivity to stressors and accompanying bouts of depression and hypersecretion of cortisol may increase across the lifespan. Furthermore, the magnitude of the stressors needed to initiate a bout of depression may become less and less until no stressor is needed to initiate the depression accompanied by hypercortisolism (Gold et al., in press). Chrousos and colleagues (Chrousos et al., 1987) suggest that the findings relating early losses, susceptibility to stressors, and adrenal activation, taken together, help integrate psychodynamic theories involving early losses and current findings involving external stressors and internal response to stressors.

Finally, a new line of evidence suggests links between hypercortisolism, psychiatric disorders and structural changes in the adrenal cortex. Adrenal weight has been found to be significantly higher in victims of violent suicide than in subjects who died of other causes (Dorovini-Zis & Zis, 1987). Because many suicide victims are depressed, it is suggested that the hyperstimulation of the adrenal cortex by ACTH leads to hypertrophy of the adrenal glands.

A critical question in the pathophysiology of psychiatric disorders is the causal direction between abnormalities in HPA functioning and gonadal functioning, especially in psychiatric disorders, such as anorexia nervosa. Based on existing literature, one might be inclined to conclude that treatment of psychiatric disorders should lead to normalization of the HPA axis functioning, which, in turn, should result in a return to adequate gonadal functioning. Very recent evidence supports at least part of such a conclusion (i.e., that treatment of depression leads to a return to normal adrenal functioning). Depressed patients, compared to normal individuals, are reported to have increased 24-hour mean plasma cortisol levels, an increased frequency of cortisol secretory episodes, and a decreased relative amplitude of cortisol circadian rhythm (Linkowski et al., 1986). After treatment either with electroconvulsive therapy or an antidepressant, cortisol concentration returned to normal and the 24-hour mean cortisol levels became similar to those of normal individuals. No comparable findings are available to link the onset of hypercortisolism attendant to clinical depression to environmental stressors.

SUMMARY AND CONCLUSIONS

Although diverse disciplines focus on the multiple causes and sequelae of stress and development, a systematic examination of the mechanisms involved in moderating stress on development has begun only recently. Recent advances based on studies of the mechanisms of physical and emotional stress (Chrousos, Loriaux, & Gold, in press) have identified both stress-related physiological structures and functions and environmental contexts that may alter the course of behavioral development. In this chapter, we discussed findings on socio-emotional stress, physical exercise stress, and stress involved in psychiatric disorders. We suggest that the physiological changes that accompany these stressors may have long-term implications for behavioral development. Although the effects of these stressors may appear to be short-term, their long-term effects may be substantial. The stress response that accompanies physical exercise, for instance, activates the adrenal axis and suppresses the gonadal axis, potentially impacting on growth and reproduction. It is important to note, however, that the models used to conceptualize physical environmental stressors and behavioral development have been developed primarily in nonhuman species. As the application of these models in research on stress and behavioral development in humans has begun only recently, our conclusions should be viewed as tentative and serve to stimulate hypothesis formation and future research.

REFERENCES

Anisman, H., & Lapierre, Y. D. (1982). Neurochemical aspects of stress and depression: Formulations and Caveats. In R. W. J. Neufeld (Ed.), *Psychological stress and psychopathology* (pp. 179–217). New York: McGraw–Hill.

Blyth, D. A., Simmons, R. G., Bulcroft, R., Felt, D., VanCleave, E. F., & Bush, D. M. (1981). The effects of physical development on self–image and satisfaction with body–image for early adolescent males. In R. G. Simmons (Ed.), *Research in community and mental health* (pp. 43–73). Greenwich, CT: JAI Press.

Britton, D. R., Koob, G. F., Rivier, J., & Vale, W. (1982). Intraventricular cortiocotropin–releasing factor enhances behavioral effects of novelty. *Life Science, 31*, 363–367.

Brooks-Gunn, J. (1987). Pubertal processes and girls' psychological adaptation. In R. M. Lerner & T. T. Foch (Eds.), *Biological-psychosocial interactions in early adolescence* (pp. 123–153). Hillsdale, NJ: Lawrence Erlbaum Associates.

Brooks-Gunn, J., & Warren, M. P. (1985). Effects of delayed menarche in different contexts: Dance and nondance students. *Journal of Youth and Adolescence, 14*, 285–300.

Brooks-Gunn, J., & Warren, M. P. (in press). Biological and social contributions to negative affect in young adolescent girls. *Child Development.*

Brown, M. R., Fisher, L. A., Spiess, J., Rivier, C., Rivier, J., & Vale, W. (1982).

Corticotropin releasing factor: Actions on the sympathetic nervous system and metabolism. *Endocrinology, 111*, 928–931.

Calogero, A. E., Gallucci, W. T., Gold, P. W., & Chrousos, G. P. (1988a). Multiple feedback regulatory loops upon rat hypothalamic corticotropin-releasing hormone secretion. Potential clinical implications. *The Journal of Clinical Investigation, 82*, 767–774.

Calogero, A. E., Gallucci, W. T., Gold, P. W., & Chrousos, G. P. (1988b). Catecholamine effects upon rat hypothalamic corticotropin-releasing hormone secretion in vitro. *The Journal of Clinical Investigation, 82*, 839–846.

Cannon, W. B. (1929). *Bodily changes in pain, hunger, fear, and rage*. Boston: Branford.

Carlson, G. A., & Cantwell, D. P. (1978). A survey of depressive symptoms, syndrome and disorder in a child psychiatric population. *Journal of Child Psychology and Psychiatry, 21*, 19–25.

Charpenet, G., Tache, Y., Forest, M. G., Haour, F., Saez, J. M., & Bernier, M. (1981). Effects of chronic intermittent immobilization stress on rat testicular androgenic function. *Endocrinology, 109*, 1254–1258.

Chrousos, G. P., Luger, A., Avgerinos, P. C., Kling, M. A., Oldfield, E. H., Nieman, L. K., Schurmeyer, T., Loriaux, D. L., & Gold, P. W. (1987). Corticotropin releasing hormone: Relevance to human physiology and pathophysiology. In R. D'Agata & G. P. Chrousos (Eds.), *Recent advances in adrenal regulation and function* (pp. 121–135). New York: Raven Press.

Chrousos, G. P., Loriaux, D. L., & Gold, P. W. (in press). *Physical and emotional stress: Biochemical mechanisms and clinical implications*, New York: Plenum.

Coe, C. L., Wiener, S. G., Rosenberg, L. T., & Levine, S. (1985). Endocrine and immune responses to separation and maternal loss in nonhuman primates. In M. Reite & T. Field (Eds.), *The psychobiology of attachment and separation* (pp. 163–199). Orlando: Academic Press.

Coe, C. L., Wiener, S. G., & Levine, S. (1983). Psychoendocrine responses of mother and infant monkeys to disturbance and separation. In L. A. Rosenblum and H. Moltz (Eds.), *Symbiosis in parent–offspring interactions* (pp. 189–214). New York: Plenum.

Collu, R., Gibb, W., & Ducharme, J. R. (1984). Effects of stress on gonadal function. *Journal of Endocrinological Investigation, 7*, 529–537.

Cumming, D. C., Quigley, M. E., & Yen, S. S. C. (1983). Acute suppression of circulating testosterone levels by cortisol in men. *Journal of Clinical Endocrinology and Metabolism, 57*, 671–673.

Dessypris, A., Kuoppasalmi, K., & Adlercreutz, H. (1976). Plasma cortisol, testosterone, androstenedione and luteinizing hormone (LH) in a non–competitive marathon run. *Journal of Steroid Biochemistry, 7*, 33–37.

Dorovini-Zis, K., & Zis, A. P. (1987). Increased adrenal weight in victims of violent suicide. *American Journal of Psychiatry, 144*, 1214–1215.

Francis, D. T. (1981). The relationship between high and low trait psychological stress, serum testosterone, and serum cortisol. *Experientia, 37*, 1296–1297.

Glickman, S. E., Frank, L. G., Davidson, J. M., Smith, E. R., & Siiteri, P. K. (1987). Androstenedione may organize or activate sex-reversed traits in female spotted hyenas. *Proceedings of the National Academy of Science, 84*, 3444–3447.

Gold, P. W., & Chrousos, G. P. (1985). Clinical studies with corticotropin releasing factor: Implications for the diagnosis and pathophysiology of depression, Cushing's Disease, and adrenal insufficiency. *Psychoneuroendocrinology, 10*, 401–419.

Gold, P. W., Goodwin, F., & Chrousos, G. P. (in press). Clinical and biochemical manifestations of depression: Relationship to the neurobiology of stress. *New England Journal of Medicine.*

Gold, P. W., Gwirtsman, H., Avgerinos, P. C., Nieman, L., Gallucci, W. T., Kaye, W., Jimerson, D., Ebert, M., Rittmaster, R. W., Loriaux, D. L., & Chrousos, G. P. (1986). Abnormal hypothalamic-pituitary-adrenal function in anorexia nervosa: Pathophysiological mechanisms in underweight and weight-corrected patients. *New England Journal of Medicine, 314,* 1335–1342.

Gold, P. W., Loriaux, D. L., Roy, A., Kling, M. A., Calabrese, J. R., Kellner, C. H., Post, R. M., Pickar, D., Galluci, W. T., Avgerinos, P. C., Paul, S., Oldfield, E. H., Cutler, G. B., Jr., & Chrousos, G. P. (1986). Responses to corticotropin-releasing hormone in the hypercortisolism of depression and Cushing's disease. *New England Journal of Medicine, 314,* 1329–1335.

Hamburg, B. A. (1974). Early adolescence: A specific and stressful stage of the life cycle. In G. Coelho, D. A. Hamburg, & J. E. Adams (Eds.), *Coping and adaptation* (pp. 101–124). New York: Basic Books.

Kagan, J., Resnick, A., & Snidman, N. (1987). The physiology and psychology of behavioral inhibition in children. *Child Development, 58,* 1459–1473.

Krulich, L., Hefco, E., Illner, P., & Read, C. B. (1974). The effects of acute stress on the secretion of LH, FSH, prolactin and GH in the normal male rat, with comments on their statistical evaluation. *Neuroendocrinology, 16,* 293–311.

Levine, S. (1984). A psychobiological approach to the ontogeny of coping. In N. Garmezy & M. Rutter (Eds.), *Stress, coping, and development in children* (pp. 107–131). New York: McGraw-Hill.

Levine, S., Coe, C. L., Smotherman, W. P., & Kaplan, J. N. (1978). Prolonged cortisol elevation in the infant squirrel monkey after reunion with mother. *Physiology & Behavior, 20,* 7–20.

Linkowski, P., Mendlewicz, J., Kerkhofs, M., Leclercq, R., Goldstein, J., Brasseur, M., Copinschi, G., & Van Cauter, E. (1986). 24-hour profiles of adrenocorticotropin, cortisol, and growth hormone in major depressive illness: Effect of antidepressant treatment. *Journal of Clinical Endocrinology and Metabolism, 65,* 141–152.

Luger, A., Deuster, P. A., Kyle, S. B., Gallucci, W. T., Montgomery, L, C., Gold, P. W., Loriaux, D. L., & Chrousos, G. P. (1987). Acute hypothalamic-pituitary-adrenal responses to the stress of treadmill exercise. *New England Journal of Medicine, 316,* 1309–1315.

MacConnie, S. E., Barkan, A., Lampman, R. M., Schork, M. A., & Beitins, I. Z. (1986). Decreased hypothalamic gonadotropin releasing hormones secretion in male marathon runners. *New England Journal of Medicine, 315,* 411–417.

Marshall, W. A., & Tanner, J. M. (1969). Variations in the pattern of pubertal changes in girls. *Archives of Disease in Children, 44,* 291–303.

Marshall, W. A., & Tanner, J. M. (1970). Variations in the pattern of pubertal changes in boys. *Archives of Disease in Children, 45,* 13–23.

Mason, J. W. (1968). A review of psychoendocrine research on the pituitary-adrenal cortical system. *Psychosomatic Medicine, 30,* 576–608.

Munck, A., Guyre, P. M., & Holbrook, N. J. (1984). Physiological functions of glucocorticoids in stress and their relation to pharmacological actions. *Endocrine Reviews, 5,* 25–44.

Nottelmann, E. D. (1982, March). Children's adjustment in school: The interaction of physical maturity and school transition. In B. Mackenzie-Haslam (Chair), *Individual differences and school structures affecting the school transitions of early adolescents.* Symposium conducted at the annual meeting of the American Educational Research Association. New York. (ERIC Document Reproduction Service No. PS 012808).

Nottelmann, E. D., Inoff-Germain, G., Susman, E. J., & Chrousos, G. P. (in press). Hormones and behavior at puberty. In J. Bancroft (Ed.), *Adolescents and puberty.* London: Oxford University Press.

Nottelmann, E. D., Susman, E. J., Inoff-Germain, G., Cutler, G. B., Jr., Loriaux, D. L., & Chrousos, G. P. (1987). Developmental processes in early adolescence: Relations between adolescent adjustment problems and chronological age, pubertal stage, and puberty-related serum hormone levels. *Journal of Pediatrics, 110,* 473–480.

Olster, D. H., & Ferin, M. (1987). Corticotropin–releasing hormone inhibits gonadatropin secretion in the ovariectomized rhesus monkey. *Journal of Clinical Endocrinology and Metabolism, 65,* 262–267.

Olweus, D. (1986). Aggression and hormones: Behavioral relationships with testosterone and adrenaline. In D. Olweus, J. Block, & M. Radke-Yarrow, (Eds.), *Development of antisocial and prosocial behavior: Research, theories, and issues* (pp. 51–72). Orlando: Academic Press.

Parker, L. N., Levin, E. R., & Lifrak, E. T. (1985). Evidence for adrenocortical adaptation to severe illness. *Journal of Clinical Endocrinology and Metabolism, 60,* 947–962.

Petersen, A. C. (1987). The nature of biological–psychological interactions: The sample case of early adolescence. In R. M. Lerner & T. T. Foch (Eds.), *Biological-psychosocial interactions in early adolescence* (pp. 35–61). Hillsdale, NJ: Lawrence Erlbaum Associates.

Petersen, A. C., & Taylor, B. (1980). The biological approach to adolescence: Biological change and psychosocial adaptation. In J. Adelson (Ed.), *Handbook of the psychology of adolescence* (pp. 115–155). New York: Wiley.

Plomin, R., & Stocker, C. (in press). Behavioral genetics and emotionality. In J. S. Reznick (Ed.), *Perspectives in behavioral inhibition.* Chicago: University of Chicago Press.

Rivier, C., & Vale, W. (1984). Influence of corticotropin-releasing factor on reproductive functions in the rat. *Endocrinology, 114,* 914–921.

Rivier, C., & Vale, W. (1985). Effect of the long-term administration of corticotropin-releasing factor on the pituitary-adrenal and pituitary-gonadal axis in the male rat. *Journal of Clinical Investigation, 75,* 689–694.

Rose, R. M. (1980). Endocrine responses to stressful psychological events. Advances in psychoneuroendcrinology. *Psychiatric Clinics of North America, 3,* 251–276.

Rutter, M., Graham, P., Chadwick, O., & Yule, W. (1976). Adolescent turmoil: Fact or fiction? *Journal of Child Psychology and Psychiatry, 17,* 35–56.

Sakakura, M., Takebe, K., & Nakagawa, S. (1975). Inhibition of luteinizing hormone secretion induced by synthetic LRH by long-term treatment with glucocorticoids in human subjects. *Journal of Clinical Endocrinology and Metabolism, 40,* 774–779.

Schaison, G., Durand, F. & Mowszowicz, I. (1978). Effect of glucocorticoids on plasma testosterone in men. *Acta Endocrinologica, 89,* 126–131.

Selye, H. (1950). *Stress: The physiology and pathology of exposure to stress.* Montreal: Acta Medical Publishers.

Sowers, J. R., Rice, B. F., & Blanchard, S. (1979). Effect of dexamethasone on luteinizing hormone and follicle stimulating hormone responses to LHRH and to clomiphene in the follicular phase of women with normal menstrual cycles. *Hormone and Metabolic Research, 11,* 478–480.

Suomi, S. J. (1984). New studies of social development in rhesus monkeys. *Verh. Dtsch. Zool. Ges, 77,* 37–44.

Suomi, S. J. (1987). Genetic and maternal contributions to individual differences in rhesus monkey biobehavioral development. In N. Krasnagor (Ed.), *Psychobiological aspects of behavioral development* (pp. 397–420). New York: Academic Press.

Susman, E. J., Nottelmann, E. D., Inoff–Germain, G., Dorn, L. D., Cutler, G. B., Jr., Loriaux, D. L., & Chrousos, G. P. (1985). The relation of relative hormonal levels and physical development and social–emotional behavior in young adolescents. *Journal of Youth and Adolescence, 14,* 245–264.

Susman, E. J., Inoff-Germain, G., Nottelmann, E. D., Loriaux, D. L., Cutler, G. B., Jr. & Chrousos, G. P. (1987). Hormones, emotional dispositions, and aggressive attributes in young adolescents. *Child Development, 58,* 1114–1134.

Susman, E. J., Nottelmann, E. D., Inoff-Germain, G.3, Dorn, L. D., & Chrousos, G. P. (in press). Physiological and behavioral aspects of stress in adolescence. In G. P. Chrousos, D. L. Loriaux, & P. W. Gold (Eds.), *Physical and emotional stress: Biochemical mechanisms and clinical implications.* New York: Plenum.

Sutton, R. E., Koob, G. F., LeMoal, M., Rivier, J., & Vale, W. (1982). Corticotropin releasing factor produces behavioral activation in rats. *Nature, 297,* 331–333.

Thomas, A., Chess, S., & Korn, S. J. (1982). The reality of difficult temperament. *Merrill–Palmer Quarterly, 28,* 1–20.

Thomas, E. B., Levine, S., & Arnold, W. J. (1968). Effects of maternal deprivation and incubation rearing upon adrenocortical activity in the adult rat. *Developmental Psychobiology, 1,* 21–29.

Valentino, R. J., Foote, S. L., & Aston-Jones, G. (1983). Corticotropin releasing factor activates noradrenergic neurons of the locus coeruleus. *Brain Research, 270,* 363–367.

Warren, M. P. (1980). The effects of exercise on pubertal progression and reproductive function in girls. *Journal of Clinical Endocrinology and Metabolism, 51,* 1150–1157.

Warren, M. P., Brooks–Gunn, J., Hamilton, L. H., Hamilton, W. G., & Warren, L. F. (1986). Scoliosis and fractures in young ballet dancers: Relation to delayed menarcheal age and secondary amenorrhea. *New England Journal of Medicine, 314,* 1348–1353.

Williams, R. B., Jr. (1986). Patterns of reactivity and stress. In K. A. Mathews, S. M. Weiss, S. B. Manuck, & R. B. Williams, Jr. (Eds.), *Handbook of stress, reactivity, and cardiovascular disease* (pp. 109–125), New York: Wiley.

3

The Sympathoadrenal System and Homeostasis: *Coping With Changes in the Internal and External Environment*

Lewis Landsberg, M.D.
Diane R. Krieger, M.D.
Beth Israel Hospital and Harvard Medical School

> *This kind of independence shown by the organism in the external environment comes from the fact that, in the living being, the tissues are, in reality, removed from direct external influences and protected by a true internal environment (milieu interieur) mostly constituted by the fluid circulating in the body.*
> *The constancy of the internal environment is the condition for free and independent life, the mechanism that makes it possible is that which assures the maintenance within the internal environment of all the conditions necessary for . . . life . . . . The constancy of the environment presupposes a perfection of the organism such that external variations are at every instant compensated and brought into balance. The conditions necessary for the life of the elements which must be brought together and maintained constant in the internal environment, for the exercise of free life, are those that we know already: water, oxygen, heat, and chemical substances or reserves.*
> *These are the same conditions as those which are necessary for life in the simple beings, except in the more perfect animals with independent life the nervous system is called upon to regulate the harmony among all these conditions.*
>
> —Claude Bernard, 1857, 1878 (Langley, 1973)

> *Biologists have long been impressed by the ability of living beings to maintain their own stability . . . . The coordinated physiological reactions which maintain most of the steady states in the body are so complex, and are so peculiar to the living organism, that it has been*

> *suggested that a specific designation for these states be employed—homeostasis.*
> *The homeostatic regulators act automatically . . . . Commonly the autonomic system, or that system in cooperation with endocrine organs, is called into action. Illustrations of these facts are seen in the . . . sympathico-adrenal influences on the glycemic level, . . . and sympathetic effects on the heart rate and . . . on blood vessels during vigorous muscular effort, and the sympathico-adrenal functions in accelerating heat production when the body temperature tends to fall.*
>
> —Walter B. Cannon, 1929 (Langley, 1973)

The concepts of a stable *internal environment* and *homeostasis* encompass modern biomedical thought and current clinical practice. The powerful influence of these concepts is, in fact, reflected in the popular recognition and acceptance of these ideas. The notion of constancy in the internal environment is generally attributed to Claude Bernard (Robin, 1979) the renowned French physiologist who recognized the need for physiological mechanisms to compensate for internal changes induced by alterations in the external world. It was the pioneering work of Walter B. Cannon, professor of physiology at the Harvard Medical School during the first half of the 20th century, however, that established the physiological basis of *homeostasis* and identified the important role played by catecholamines in the regulation of many processes that contribute to a stable internal environment (Cannon, 1939; Langley, 1973).

Simply stated *homeostasis* refers to both the stability of the internal environment and the physiological processes involved in the maintenance of that stability. Working in concert, the endocrine system and the autonomic nervous system regulate a multiplicity of processes that preserve the constancy of the internal environment. These physiological processes, evolved to defend the internal environment in the face of external challenge, endow the mammalian organism with a remarkable capability to resist internal disruption despite marked changes in the external environment. This chapter addresses the role played by the sympathoadrenal system in the maintenance of homeostasis.

The functional state of the sympathetic nerves and adrenal medulla is directly dependent on regulatory centers within the brain. Input from the cerebral cortex and the limbic system serves to coordinate autonomic activity with cognitive processes and emotional reactions by influencing the activity of the regulatory brainstem centers that initiate sympathoadrenal outflow. These connections play an important physiological role, as described here, in that they prepare an organism to withstand a physiological challenge in anticipation of the acute event. Under certain circumstances, however, recruitment of a sympathoadrenal response may occur in response to perceived threat but in the absence of an appropriate physiological outlet; in situations such as these the resulting physiological changes may be detrimental. These concepts are clarified in this chapter with specific examples. Before proceeding, however, it is necessary to consider the organization of the sympathoadrenal system and methods of assessing sympathoadrenal activity.

ORGANIZATION OF THE SYMPATHOADRENAL SYSTEM

The sympathetic nervous system and the adrenal medulla form an integrated functional unit referred to as the *sympathoadrenal system*. Catecholamine release at sympathetic nerve endings and from the adrenal medulla is the direct result of a descending flow of impulse traffic originating in regulatory centers in the hypothalamus, pons, and medulla oblongata. Bulbospinal tracts from these regulatory centers descend in the spinal cord and synapse with typical preganglionic cholinergic neurons in the intermediolateral cell column of the spinal cord. These preganglionic axons exit the spinal cord and either (a) synapse with postganglionic sympathetic neurons in the paravertebral sympathetic ganglia; (b) pass through the sympathetic ganglia, collect as the splanchnic nerves, and synapse with postganglionic sympathetic neurons in the preoaortic abdominal ganglia; or (c) innervate directly the endocrine secretory (chromaffin) cells of the adrenal medulla. The innervation of the adrenal medulla is thus analogous to that of the postganglionic sympathetic neurons. The secretory product of the adrenal medulla (epinephrine) is secreted into the bloodstream. Postganglionic neurons, located in the peripheral sympathetic ganglia, give rise to axons that are widely distributed throughout the organ systems where they innervate vascular and visceral smooth muscle and endocrine and exocrine glands. In peripheral tissues the terminal sympathetic fibers ramify extensively to form a ground plexus or syncitial network that establishes intimate contact between the nerve endings and effector cells.

Norepinephrine (NE) is the adrenergic neurotransmitter; it is released in response to nerve impulses invading the terminal sympathetic fibers and exerts its physiologic effect locally, in the immediate vicinity of release. Epinephrine (E) is released from the adrenal medulla and distributed via the circulation to tissues throughout the body. Both NE and E influence physiological processes by interacting with adrenergic receptors on effector cells. Two major categories of adrenergic receptor (alpha and beta) are recognized: representative responses mediated by the alpha-receptor include vasoconstriction, pupillary dilation, and intestinal relaxation while the beta-receptor mediates cardiac stimulation, increase in metabolic rate, and substrate mobilization (lipolysis, glycogenolysis, and gluconeogenesis). Although a variety of factors have been identified that modify the sensitivity of effector tissues to catecholamines (some, but not all, mediated via changes in adrenergic receptors), the level of activity, or functional state, of the sympathoadrenal system appears to be the major determinant of the physiological response under most circumstances. Similarly, although a variety of mediators are known to influence the relationship between transmitter release and nerve impulse traffic within the peripheral sympathetic nervous system (prejunctional or presynaptic modulators) the activity of the sympathetic nervous system appears (in most circumstances) to have overriding importance in establishing most physiological responses. The assessment of sympathoadrenal activity, therefore, becomes critical in establishing the role played by catecholamines in the maintenance of homeostasis.

Generalized Versus Discriminating Responses

Although it is common to think of generalized sympathetic responses as emobied in the "fight or flight" response of Cannon (1939), the recent application of sophisticated techniques has demonstrated that the distribution of sympathetic outflow is nonhomogeneous. Depending on the physiological situation, sympathetic activity may be increased in some organ systems but not in others (Landsberg & Young, 1986). Similarly, the relationship between sympathetic nervous system responses and those of the adrenal medulla is complex (Young & Landsberg, 1980). The traditional view, enunciated by Cannon, holds that the sympathetic nerves and adrenal medulla work in concert, with bloodborne catecholamines from the adrenal medulla reinforcing the physiologic effect of sympathetic neuronal stimulation. It is clear from recent studies, however, that in several physiological situations the adrenal medulla is stimulated when the sympathetic nervous system is suppressed (Young, Rosa, & Landsberg, 1984). An important role for the adrenal medulla, therefore, may be the provision of catecholamines during periods of sympathetic nervous system suppression. Thus, although sympathetic nervous system and adrenal medullary responses are always highly coordinated, the two major limbs of the sympathoadrenal system are not always activated at the same time. The response, rather, is tailored to the physiological requirements and the needs of the organism as a whole.

Direct and Indirect Effects

In addition to the direct stimulation of various processes, catecholamines influence the secretion of endocrine glands and the distribution of blood flow. Direct effects of catecholamines are those induced by the interactions of catecholamines with adrenergic receptors on effector cells. Stimulation of arteriolar vasoconstriction and activation of hormone sensitive triglyceride lipase in adipose tissue are examples of the direct effect of alpha- and beta-receptor stimulation, respectively. Indirect effects of catecholamines are those induced by changes in the secretion of other hormones or by alterations in blood flow. Generally, the indirect effects of catecholamines enhance the direct effects by creating the proper hormonal and circulatory milieu for the full expression of the stimulated process. In addition to directly stimulating arteriolar smooth muscle, for example, catecholamines stimulate the release of renin from the kidney. Renin increases the concentration of angiotensin in the circulation that also increases arteriolar vasoconstriction and potentiates the effects of catecholamines. Similarly, under certain circumstances, catecholamines suppress insulin release. Insulin exerts an inhibitory effect on hormone sensitive triglyceride lipase so that the suppression of insulin by catecholamines enhances the direct effect of catecholamines on triglyceride lipase and fosters lipolysis. Examples of these interactions in different physiologic and pathophysiologic states are given later.

The Peripheral Dopaminergic System

In addition to the classic sympathoadrenal system, recent work has demonstrated the existence of a peripheral dopaminergic system. The structural organization of this system, however, has just begun to emerge and may involve, to a considerable extent, the decarboxylation of circulating dopa to dopamine (DA) in peripheral effector tissues with the local generation of a physiological response (Williams et al., 1986).

ASSESSMENT OF SYMPATHOADRENAL ACTIVITY

The assessment of sympathoadrenal activity is confounded by several unique problems. In general, the effects of catecholamines are induced rapidly and dissipated quickly, unlike the slower, more prolonged effects of other hormones. The plasma half life of catecholamines is short, generally under 2 minutes, as a consequence of extensive metabolism in peripheral tissues and uptake into sympathetic nerve endings. The acquisition of the plasma sample, furthermore, may be associated with significant activation of the sympathoadrenal system necessitating careful attention to the state of the subject at the time the plasma sample is acquired. By convention, basal catecholamine levels are obtained after the subject has rested supine in a relaxed environment for 30 minutes and the sample withdrawn from a previously placed indwelling intravenous line. This presents a particular problem in experiments involving small animals because chronic instrumentation is required to get meaningful values. Assessing sympathetic activity is further confounded by the fact that norepinephrine is a neurotransmitter rather than a circulating hormone; under most circumstances circulating levels of NE are below the threshhold for stimulation of adrenergic receptors (Silverberg, Shah, Haymond, & Cryer, 1978). Epinephrine, in contrast, circulates at levels that stimulate adrenergic receptors (Clutter, Bier, Shah, & Cryer, 1980) in spite of the fact that the actual concentration of epinephrine in plasma is, on the average, considerably lower than that of NE.

Limitations of Plasma and Urinary Measurements

Adrenal Medullary Activity. Because E is the hormone of the adrenal medulla, the functional state should be reflected in plasma levels and urinary excretion. In general this is the case; elevated plasma levels of E are associated with adrenal medullary activation and urinary E excretion provides an integrated measure of adrenal medullary secretion over time. Venous plasma levels of E, however, provide a relatively insensitive index of adrenal medullary activity. The venous level of E is considerably lower (40%–50%) than the arterial (Halter, Pflug, & Tolas, 1980; Hjemdahl, 1986; Joyce, Beilin, Vandongen, & Davidson, 1982) reflecting uptake and metabolism of E by the tissues (hind or forelimb) giving rise to the venous drainage that is sampled. The fractional extraction of E, moreover, is not constant and appears to vary widely in different physiological states depending, importantly, on bloodflow. Thus, arterial samples, or arterialized venous blood gives a more sensitive index of adrenal medullary activity than do venous levels.

Under certain circumstances, in experimental animals, adrenal medullary E depletion occurs when adrenal medullary activity is markedly increased. Under these circumstances measurement of adrenal medullary epinephrine content may serve as an index of adrenal medullary activation (Young, Fish, & Landsberg, 1983; Young & Landsberg, 1979a).

Sympathetic Nervous System Activity. The assessment of sympathetic nervous system activity from measurements of NE in plasma and urine is confounded by a variety of factors including the following: (a) NE is a neurotransmitter and not a circulating hormone; the level of NE in the plasma reflects overflow from adrenergic synapses throughout the body and is only tangentially related to NE release from sympathetic nerve endings. Well-documented sympathetic stimulation has been noted in the absence of significant changes in circulating NE (Cryer, Haymond, Santiago, & Shah, 1976). (b) The plasma half life of NE is brief and the plasma clearance is influenced by changes in sympathetic activity (Esler et al., 1984). Increased sympathetic activity is associated with enhanced plasma clearance while, conversely, diminished sympathetic activity slows the plasma clearance rate. These alterations decrease the sensitivity of plasma NE measurements as a measure of sympathetic activity. (c) The dissociation of sympathetic nervous system and adrenal medullary activity, under certain circumstances, invalidates the use of plasma and urinary NE determinations as indices of sympathetic nervous system activity. Under basal conditions the adrenal medullary contribution to the circulating pool of NE is trivial; when the adrenal medulla is stimulated, however, NE as well as E is secreted (Johnson, Young, & Landsberg, 1983; Landsberg, Greff, Gunn, & Young, 1980; Rappaport, Young, & Landsberg, 1982; Young et al., 1983; Young & Landsberg, 1979; Young et al., 1984). Thus, when the adrenal medulla is activated origin of NE from the sympathetic nerves cannot be inferred and plasma or urinary NE cannot be used to assess sympathetic nervous system activity. (d) Nonhomogenous sympathetic outflow, coupled with the practical requirement of sampling plasma from a peripheral limb vein limits sharply the utility of plasma measurements in the assessment of sympathetic activity in organs or locations removed from the site of sampling. In distinction to E, peripheral venous levels of NE are higher than those of arterial samples by some 20%–40% (Halter et al., 1980; Hjemdahl, 1986; Lake, Ziegler, & Kopin, 1976). Since the tissues of the limb extract NE as well as E the fact that the venous NE levels exceed the arterial means that much of the NE sampled at peripheral venous sites reflects norepinephrine release in the tissues immediately downstream from the venous sampling site (Hjemdahl, 1986). The NE content of venous blood draining a limb reflects, importantly, sympathetic activity in nerves supplying limb vasculature and skeletal muscle (Wallin et al., 1981). Although this is frequently of interest, changes in sympathetic activity at other internal sites may be poorly represented in a blood sample obtained from a limb vessel. (e) Similar considerations apply to the kidney that extensively metabolizes NE presented in the arterial circulation (Silva, Landsberg, & Besarab, 1979), and adds a nephrogenous component derived from the sympathetic innervation of the kidney. For all these reasons information about sympathetic nervous system activity from measurements of plasma and urinary NE levels is limited.

NE Turnover Measurements in the Tissues of Experimental Animals

Some of these difficulties may be overcome by the measurement of NE turnover rate in the tissues of sympathetically innervated organs of experimental animals (Landsberg & Young, 1986). Such measurements, employing either tracer doses of NE, or the inhibition of NE synthesis, permit separate independent assessment of sympathetic activity in different organs and are unaffected by changes in adrenal medullary activity. These techniques, furthermore, permit a comparison of sympathetic outflow in different tissues. Turnover measurements have been useful in studying sympathetic outflow in a variety of physiological situations relating to the maintenance of homeostasis. These techniques have been useful in elucidating the sympathoadrenal responses in several different physiologic states.

SYMPATHOADRENAL ACTIVITY IN SEVERAL DIFFERENT PHYSIOLOGICAL STATES

Cold Exposure

The sympathoadrenal system plays a critical role in the mammalian response to cold exposure (Landsberg & Young, 1985a). Experimental destruction or blockade or the sympathoadrenal system prevents the maintenance of body temperature during cold exposure and leads to death in hypothermia (Maickel, Matussek, Stern, & Brodie, 1967). Exposure to a cold environment stimulates temperature receptors in the skin and temperature sensitive neurons in the central nervous system (hypothalamus, lower brain stem, and spinal cord) generating afferent neural input that is integrated in the hypothalamus (Gale, 1973). As a consequence, sympathetic outflow, as assessed by norepinephrine turnover rates in several sympathetically innervated organ systems increases markedly (Young & Landsberg, 1979b; Young, Saville, Rothwell, Stock, & Landsberg, 1982). The increase in sympathetic outflow is sustained throughout the period of cold exposure (Landsberg, Saville, & Young, 1984). The adrenal medulla is stimulated to a much lesser degree (Young & Landsberg, 1981) and the stimulation is not sustained over time (Leduc, 1961).

The increase in sympathetic activity diminishes heat loss and increases heat production. Sympathetically mediated peripheral vasoconstriction in subcutaneous tissues converses body heat by diminishing heat loss to the environment. This is particularly important in the limbs where peripheral venoconstriction (Webb-Peploe, & Shepard, 1975) shunts blood from the superficial veins to the deeper venae comitantes that surround the major arteries supplying the limb. This results in a countercurrent heat exchange mechanism that removes heat from arterial blood perfusing the extremities, thereby antagonizing loss of heat to the environment.

Sympathetic stimulation also markedly increases metabolic heat production (Hsieh, Carlson, & Gray, 1957). In small laboratory animals, and in the neonates or virtually all mammalian species, brown adipose tissue represents the major site of catecholamine-mediated heat production (Landsberg & Young, 1983). In large adult mammals a role for brown adipose tissue has been controversial, but recent evidence (Lean, James, Jennings, & Trayhurn, 1986a, 1986b) is consistent with a role for this tissue in adult humans.

Catecholamines are also involved in mobilizing substrates as fuel sources for the increased heat production (Depocas, 1961; Maickel, Susman, Yamada, & Brodie, 1963) by stimulating lipolysis in adipose tissue and glycogenolysis in liver and muscle. These direct effects of catecholamines are reinforced by indirect effects that result from suppression of insulin (Baum & Porte, 1971) and stimulation of glucagon (Seitz, Krone, Wilke, & Tarnowski, 1981). Sympathetic stimulation of the heart supports the cardiac output that increases in direct proportion to oxygen consumption (Raven, Niki, Dahms, & Horvath, 1970) and insures adequate delivery of oxygen and substrates to metabolizing tissues.

Thus, changes in sympathoadrenal outflow subserve a complex array of physiological alterations that enable the mammalian homeotherm to maintain body temperature in the face of environmental cold.

Extracellular Fluid Volume Depletion

The sympathetic nervous system also plays a major role in the regulation of extracellular fluid volume and in the response to volume depletion. The role of the adrenal medulla is clearly secondary but in cases of severe volume depletion or hemorrhage recruitment of adrenal medullary secretion supports the effects of sympathetic stimulation, a situation simiilar to that noted in the response to cold exposure. The sympathetic nervous system is activated by a fall in venous return or by a decrease in arterial pressure. Stretch receptors in the great veins and atria (capacitance portion of the circulation) and in the aortic arch and carotid sinus (resistance portion of the circulation) are stimulated by an increase in venous or arterial pressure; impulses generated in these stretch receptors are carried back to the central nervous system in the 9th and 10th cranial nerves. Increasing impulse traffic in these pathways (increase in pressure) exerts an inhibitory effect on sympathetic outflow (Landsberg & Young, 1985a). Conversely, when venous or arterial pressure falls decreased impulse traffic from these stretch receptors results in disinhibition of central sympathetic centers and an increase in sympathetic outflow to the vasculature and kidneys. As a consequence, sympathetically mediated constriction of vascular smooth muscle increases tone in the capacitance and resistance portions of the circulation shunting blood to the heart to maintain cardiac output, and increasing peripheral resistance to maintain blood pressure. The pattern of sympathetically mediated vasoconstriction maintains blood flow to the heart and brain at the expense of other organs.

Sympathetic stimulation of the kidney in response to volume depletion (Oliver, Pinto, Sciacca, & Cannon, 1980) increases renal sodium reabsorption by direct effects on the nephron (DiBona, 1982). The direct effects of sympathetic stimulation are supported by vascular and endocrine indirect effects. Sympathetically mediated stimulation of renin release enhances angiotensin formation which potentiates sympathetically mediated vasoconstriction. Sympathetic effects on the renal vasculature also foster sodium reabsorption by redistributing renal blood flow from the cortical to the juxtamedullary nephrons and by increasing peritubular oncotic pressure (Gotshall & Itskovitz, 1977; Pomeranz, Birtch, & Barger, 1968). Activation of the renin angiotensin system also potentiates renal sodium reabsorption by stimulating the secretion of aldosterone which fosters distal tubular sodium conservation. The net result of these physiological adjustments is preservation of the circulation in the face of the challenge induced by fluid loss or hemorrhage.

Starvation and Hypoglycemia

The physiological adjustment to starvation also involves an integrated sympathoadrenal response (Landsberg & Young, 1985b). Fasting is associated with suppression of sympathetic nervous system activity (Young & Landsberg, 1977). Fasting-induced suppression of sympathetic activity appears to be secondary to a decrease in insulin mediated glucose metabolism within critical insulin-glucose sensitive neurons related to the ventromedial hypothalamus (Landsberg & Young, 1985c; Young & Landsberg, 1980). Suppressed sympathetic activity reduces metabolic rate thereby conserving calories when intake is limited. Mobilization of substrates from fuel stores, which involves lipolysis in adipose tissue and enhancement of hepatic glucose output, is stimulated by a modest concomitant increase in adrenal medullary secretion (Young et al., 1984). The increase in adrenal medullary stimulation fosters substrate mobilization since fasting enhances the sensitivity of adipose tissue to catecholamine-induced lipolysis (Arner, Engfeldt, & Nowak, 1981). The level of epinephrine achieved during fasting, however, appears to be below the threshhold for the stimulation of catecholamine mediated thermogenesis (Sjostrom et al., 1983). The pattern of suppressed sympathetic nervous system activity, along with stimulation of the adrenal medulla, thus results in diminished metabolic rate and enhanced substrate mobilization contributing importantly to the physiological adjustments associated with starvation.

The sympathoadrenal response to hypoglycemia also entails sympathetic nervous system suppression but the associated increase in adrenal medullary secretion is considerably more prominent (Landsberg et al., 1980; Rappaport et al., 1982; Young & Landsberg, 1979a). The adrenal medullary response appears to be initiated by glucose sensitive neurons within the hypothalamus, the caudal brain stem, and the spinal cord (Landsberg & Young, 1985a). The vigorous epinephrine response increases hepatic glucose output and mobilizes hepatic glucose production in response to the central nervous system glucose deficiency.

Thus, the pattern of sympathoadrenal response to starvation and hypoglycemia is substantially different than that induced by cold exposure or volume depletion. Sympathetic suppression plays a critical role in diminishing sympathetically mediated thermogenesis, whereas adrenal medullary stimulation fosters substrate mobilization.

Trauma and Hypoxia

In the experimental animal, the sympathoadrenal response to acute traumatic injury (Young et al., 1983) or to acute moderate reduction in atmospheric oxygen tension (Johnson et al., 1983) is similarly associated with sympathetic nervous system suppression and concomitant marked adrenal medullary stimulation. The afferent signals that initiate the sympathoadrenal responses in these two circumstances have not been identified with certainty. In acute trauma, a particularly abrupt decrease in venous return and cognitive factors related to the sight of blood may be involved. Presumably sympathetic suppression contributes to the decrease in metabolic rate that occurs in these situations while adrenal medullary stimulation supports the circulation and provides substrate for vital functions. In the chronic phase of both traumatic injury and hypoxic exposure, however, the sympathoadrenal response changes. In both these situations the initial suppression of sympathetic activity abates and sympathetic stimulation develops along with a diminution in adrenal medullary activity. Thus, different patterns of sympathoadrenal response develop over time in response to particular environmental challenges.

The demonstration of sympathetic nervous system suppression in the face of adrenal medullary stimulation, documented in these studies as well as in those involving fasting and hypoglycemia was made possible utilizing techniques that measure norepinephrine turnover in peripheral sympathetically innervated tissues. Adrenal medullary stimulation, which increases both epinephrine and norepinephrine secretion and elevates plasma and urinary levels of both these catecholamines renders these measurements useless in evaluating the functional state of the sympathetic nervous system.

UNIQUE ASPECTS OF SYMPATHOADRENAL REGULATION: RELATIONSHIP TO MENTAL STRESS

Role of Anticipation

In many of the physiological responses of the sympathoadrenal system previously described (see Table 3.1) distinct afferent signals that initiate the sympathoadrenal response have been identified. Thus, a fall in environmental temperature, venous return, or plasma glucose level have been shown to trigger

TABLE 3.1
Representative Physiologic Responses of the Sympathoadrenal System

External Challenge	*Sympathoadrenal Response*		*Afferent Signals*	*Direct Effects*	*Indirect Effects*		*Integrated Physiological Responses*
	SNS	*Adrenal Medulla*			*Hormonal*	*Vascular*	
Cold exposure	↑↑ Heart ↑↑↑ BAT – Liver – Kidney	± ↑	Cutaneous temperature receptors Temperature sensitive neurons (hypothalamus, spinal cord)	Subcutaneous vasoconstriction Cardiac stimulation Increased metabolic rate Increased lipolysis Increased hepatic glucose output	Decreased insulin secretion Increased glucagon secretion	Increased cardiac output Distribution of blood flow to tissues	Heat conservation Heat production Provision and delivery of substrate
Volume depletion (Fluid loss, hemorrhage)	↑↑ Heart ↑↑ Vasculature ↑↑ Kidneys ↑↑ Gut	± ↑	Stretch receptors in great veins and arteries (fall in venous return, fall in blood pressure)	Vasoconstriction Cardiac stimulation Increased renal sodium reabsorption	Increased renin secretion (increase in angiotensin and aldosterone)	Redistribution of renal bood flow (from cortex and towards medulla)	Maintenance of blood pressure and organ perfusion (particularly heart and brain) Conservation of plasma volume
Starvation	↓↓↓	↑	Decreased insulin-mediated glucose metabolism in hypothalamus	Decreased metabolic rate	Decreased peripheral conversion of thyroxine to triiodo-thyronine	Diminished vasoconstriction in adipose tissue	Decrease in energy utilization Provision of substrate for metabolism

Hypoglycemia	↓↓	↑↑↑	Decreased plasma glucose	Increased glycogenolysis in liver and muscle Increased lipolysis	Decreased insulin secretion		Restores plasma glucose Provides alternate substrate (free fatty acids)
Trauma acute	↓	↑↑↑	? Abrupt fall in venous return ? Cognitive factors	Decreased metabolic rate Increased lipolysis Increased hepatic glucose output Vasoconstriction Cardiac stimulation	Decreased insulin secretion Increased glucagon secretion		Maintenance of circulation Decrease in energy utilization Provision of substrate
Trauma chronic	↑↑	↑	?	Increased metabolic rate Increased lipolysis, hepatic glucose output	Increased glucagon secretion		Provision and delivery of substrates for healing

BAT = brown adipose tissue

the appropriate sympathoadrenal response to cold exposure, volume depletion, or hypoglycemia. These afferent signals are integrated at the level of the hypothalamus and lower brain stem and appropriate changes in central sympathoadrenal outflow initiated. Important connections, however, also exist between the regulatory brain stem sympathetic centers and the cerebral cortex and the limbic lobes. These connections serve to couple autonomic response with conscious mental processes on the one hand, and with emotional reactions on the other. These connections exert an important role in metabolic regulation and also form the basis for sympathoadrenal activation in response to a group of diverse stimuli frequently referred to as *stress*.

The relationship between cognitive processes and autonomic regulatory centers means that the sympathoadrenal system can be activated in anticipation of an environmental challenge. Prior to strenuous exercise, for example, plasma NE levels (and, as a consequence, plasma renin levels) rise in anticipation of the upcoming physical activity (Hartley et al., 1972; Mason et al., 1973). Activation of the sympathoadrenal system prior to the onset of vigorous exertion lessens the impact of the activity on the internal milieu. In the absence of this anticipatory response, increase in sympathoadrenal activity would depend on reflex activation in response to changes in the internal environment due to the exercise itself such as a fall in venous return or blood pressure. Prior activation of the sympathoadrenal system, on the other hand, brings physiologic responses into play that limit the impact of the activity on the internal environment. Thus, tachycardia, venoconstriction, enhanced renal sodium reabsorption all antagonize a fall in cardiac output at the initiation of exercise. Anticipatory increases in sympathoadrenal activity form the basis of Canon's "flight or fight" response. Perceived threat or challenge of any type, including fear or other emotional responses have a similar capacity to engage the sympathoadrenal system.

Mental or Emotional Stress

The neuroendocrine response to cognitive stress has been difficult to characterize accurately. Stress research in humans, though improved by ambulatory monitoring of plasma and vital signs, remains limited by difficulties in study design as well as the problems inherent in the interpretation of urine and plasma catecholamine measurements previously described (Dimsdale, 1984). Nonetheless, the large literature involving a variety of laboratory and field "stresses" provides some insight into the adrenal medullary and SNS responses elicited by different stressful situations ranging from monotony to extreme arousal. Great variation has been observed among individuals reacting to the same stimulus (Arnetz & Fjellner, 1986). Many factors including age, sex, and personality style all affect the individual's physiologic response to "stress" that is also influenced by the quality and intensity of the stimulus (Table 3.2).

Public speaking,a potent stimulant of fear and anxiety, has been studied

TABLE 3.2
Representative Sympathoadrenal Responses to Psychological Stimuli

Stimulus	*Medulla*	*SNS*	*Time Course*	*Peripheral Manifestation*
Fear, anxiety	↑↑	↑	Rapid return to baseline	Increased heart rate Tremor Increased platelet aggregation
Mental effort	↑↑	± during stimulus ↑ after stimulus	E sustained	Increased heart rate Increased blood pressure
Anticipation of pain, violence	↑↑	–		Decreased heart rate
Monotony	↑	↑	E increases slightly over study period NE decreases during stimulus	Decreased heart rate

E = epinephrine
NE = norepinephrine

extensively as a model of anticipation and habituation to novelty (Dimsdale & Moss, 1980a; Taggart, Carruthers, & Somerville, 1973). Increases in heart rate reach maximum levels in the moments before and 1 minute into public speaking (Moss & Wynar, 1970) and are paralleled by significant increases in E and lesser increases of NE (Dimsdale & Moss, 1980a). The E peak declines to baseline by midway into the stimulus (Dimsdale & Moss, 1980b) once uncertainty decreases. When plasma is sampled before and after, rather than during speaking, an NE response is observed without an increase in E (Taggart et al., 1973) illustrating the importance of sample timing and change in emotional state with habituation.

A more sustained adrenal medullary response is engendered by experimental tasks designed to produce intense mental effort (Akerstedt et al., 1983). In some studies blood pressure, heart rate, and E all rise and remain elevated until the task is completed; in others a more significant NE response has been noted (Dimsdale, 1984). The disparate results could reflect the great individual variation in stress responses. In one study (Akerstedt et al., 1983) NE did not rise until after mental effort ceased. The cause of this late rise in NE has not been studied and may be compensatory for BP decreases seen in the post-task period. The discordance between tachycardia and the NE levels noted in some of the studies may result from selective SNS cardiac stimulation not reflected in forearm venous blood or from effects on vagally mediated parasysmpathetic tone. Forearm blood NE levels may be further lowered by stress induced inhibition of muscle SNS activity (Akerstedt et al., 1983).

The anticipation of violence (Carruthers & Taggart, 1973) or pain (Hedgworth-Whitty, Carruthers & Gordon, 1976) also results in predominantly adrenal medullary stimulation but differs from other types of arousal in that relative bradycardia usually accompanies the rise in E (Carruthers & Taggart, 1973). This suggests an important parasympathetic response to these stimuli. The stress of understimulation, produced experimentally by monotonous tasks performed in isolation, results in both sympathetic nervous system and adrenal medullary activation (Frankenhaeuser, Nordheden, Myrsten, & Post, 1971). While most experimental stressors cause adrenal medullary stimulation, NE responses have been linked to stimuli producing hostility, aggression (Lewis, 1975), and expected outcomes (Taggart et al., 1973).

Chronic psychological stimulation in animals increases the circulatory levels of NE and E as well as the activity of the biosynthetic enzymes in the adrenal medulla, an effect thought to be neuronally mediated (Henry, Stephens, Axelrod, & Mueller, 1971). Chronic stress in humans has not been studied extensively.

The acute sympathoadrenal response to psychological stress has both homeostatic and maladaptive features. The sympathetic nervous system activation that occurs before the actual stimulus could serve to provide the necessary arousal for improved performance. The catecholamine rise during monotonous tasks has been shown to enhance performance (Frankenhaeuser et al., 1971). The experience of unpleasant palpitations associated with tachycardia, however, can feed back positively on the sympathetic nervous system and amplify the physical manifestations.

The sympathetic nervous system activation may also have a detrimental effect on patients with coronary disease. In the presence of coronary artery disease increased ventricular ectopic activity and ECG changes have been noted to accompany increases in plasma catecholamines produced by experimental psychological stress (Taggart et al., 1973).

DEVELOPMENT OF THE SYMPATHOADRENAL SYSTEM

Limited information is available about the sympathetic nervous system and adrenomedullary development in humans. The sheep adrenal medulla forms from migrating neural crest cells and is innervated by 120 days of gestation. At this early date the medulla is responsive to hypoxemic stress (Heymann, 1984). In humans adrenal medullary development is characterized by a gradual increase in the proportion of epinephrine produced compared with norepinephrine (Lewis, 1975). In early fetal life the adrenal medulla produces only norepinephrine. By birth epinephrine represents 30% of adrenal catecholamine production and increases to 59% by 2 years of age (Loggie & Van Maanen, 1972). In the neonate, insulin-induced hypoglycemia produces an epinephrine response.

The sympathetic nervous system is also incompletely developed at birth. The human heart is innervated early in development. In some species beta adrenergic influence on the fetal heart is small early in gestation. Stressful conditions, however, such as hemorrhage and hypoxemia, result in a definite increase in beta adrenergic stimulation (Heymann, 1984). Alpha adrenergic responses make a progressive contribution to vascular tone throughout fetal life. It has been suggested that the norepinephrine from the adrenal and fetal paraaortic bodies (extra adrenal chromaffin cells) supports vascular tone until the sympathetic nervous system takes over (Lewis, 1975). Adrenergic receptors, though functional at gestation, increase in concentration and responsiveness in early infancy (Heymann, 1984). Recent evidence suggests that diminished norepinephrine-induced lipolysis in the first year of life is due, in part, to enhanced alpha inhibition of lipolysis in infants (Marcus, Karpe, Bolme, Sonnenfeld, & Arner, 1987). This limitation of lipolysis may have a protective effect during early life. The cold pressor and tilt table responses of neonates resemble those of the adult (Loggie & Van Maaen, 1972).

REFERENCES

Akerstedt, T., Gillberg, M., Hjemdahl, P., Sigurdson, K., Gustavsson, I., Daleskog, M., & Pollare, T. (1983). Comparison of urinary and plasma catecholamine responses to mental stress. *Acta Physiologica Scandinavica, 117*, 19–26.

Arner, P., Engfeldt, P., & Nowak, J. (1981). In vivo observation on the lipolytic effect of noradrenaline during therapeutic fasting. *Journal of Clinical Endocrinology and Metabolism, 53*, 1207–1212.

Arnetz, B. B., & Fjellner, B. (1986). Psychological predictors of neuro-endocrine responses to mental stress. *Journal of Psychosomatic Research, 30*(3), 297–305.

Baum, D., & Porte, D. (1971). Alpha-adrenergic inhibition of immunoreactive insulin release during deep hypothermia. *American Journal of Physiology, 221*, 303–311.

Cannon, W. B. (1939). *The wisdom of the body.* New York: Norton.

Carruthers, M., & Taggart, P. (1973). Vagotonicity of violence; biochemical and cardiac responses to violent films and television programmes. *British Medical Journal, 3*, 384–389.

Clutter, W. E., Bier, D. M., Shah, S. D., & Cryer, P. E. (1980). Epinephrine plasma metabolic clearance rates and physiologic thresholds for metabolic and hemodynamic actions in man. *Journal of Clinical Investigation, 66*, 94–101.

Cryer, P. E., Haymond, N. W., Santiago, J. V., & Shah, S. D. (1976). Norepinephrine and epinephrine release and adrenergic mediation of smoking-associated hemodynamic and metabolic events. *New England Journal of Medicine, 295*, 573–577.

Depocas, F. (1961). Biochemical changes in exposure and acclimation to cold environments. *British Medical Bulletin, 17*, 25–31.

DiBona, G. F. (1982). Neural mechanisms in body fluid homeostasis. *Federal Proceedings, 45*, 2871–2884.

Dimsdale, J. E. (1984). Generalizing from laboratory studies of field studies of human stress physiology. *Psychosomatic Medicine, 46*(5), 463–469.

Dimsdale, J. E., & Moss, J. (1980a). Plasma catecholamines in stress and exercise. *Journal of the American Medical Association, 243*(4), 340–342.

Dimsdale, J. E., & Moss, J. (1980b). Short-term catecholamine response to psychological stress. *Psychosomatic Medicine, 42*(5), 493–497.

Esler, M., Jennings, G., Korner, P., Blomberg, P., Sacharias, N., & Leonard, P. (1984). Measurement of total, and organ-specific, nonadrenaline kinetics in humans. *American Journal of Physiology, 247*, E21-E28.

Frankenhaeuser, M., Nordheden, B., Myrsten, A-L., & Post, B. (1971). Psychophysiological reactions to understimulation and overstimulation. *Acta Physiologica Scandinavica, 35*, 298–308.

Gale, C. C. (1973). Neuroendocrine aspects of thermoregulation. *Annual Review of Physiology, 35*, 391–430.

Gotshall, R. W., & Itskovitz, H. D. (1977). Redistribution of renal cortical blood flow by renal nerve stimulation and norepinephrine infusion. *Proceedings of the Society for Experimental Biology and Medicine, 154*, 60–63.

Halter, J. B., Pflug, E. A., & Tolas, A. G. (1980). Arterial-venous differences of plasma catecholamines in man. *Metabolism, 29*, 9–12.

Hartley, L. H., Mason, J. W., Hogan, R. P., Jones, L. G., Kotchen, T. A., Mougey, E. H., Wherry, F. E., Pennington, L. L., & Ricketts, P. T. (1972). Multiple hormonal responses to prolonged exercise in relation to physical training. *Journal of Applied Physiology, 33*, 607–610.

Henry, J. P., Stephens, P. M., Axelrod, J., & Mueller, R. A. (1971). Effect of psychosocial stimulation on the enzymes involved in the biosynthesis and metabolism of noradrenaline and adrenaline. *Psychosomatic Medicine, 33*(3), 227–237.

Heymann, M. A., (1984). Biophysical evaluation of fetal status: fetal cardiovascular physiology. In R. K. Creasy & R. Resnik (Eds.), *Maternal-fetal medicine* (pp. 259–274). Philadelphia, PA: Saunders.

Hjemdahl, P. (1986). Measurements of plasma catecholamines by HPLC and the relation of their concentrations to sympathoadrenal activity. In M. H. Joseph, M. Fillenz, I. A. Macdonald, & C. A. Marsden (Eds.), *Monitoring neurotransmitter release during behaviour* (pp. 17–32). Chichester, England: Ellis Horwood Ltd.

Hsieh, A. C. L., Carlson, L. D., & Gray, G. (1957). Role of the sympathetic nervous system in the control of chemical regulation of heat production. *American Journal of Physiology, 190*, 247–251.

Johnson, T. S, Young, J. B., & Landsberg, L. (1983). Sympathoadrenal responses to acute and chronic hypoxia in the rat. *Journal of Clinical Investigation, 71*, 1263–1272.

Joyce, D. A., Beilin, L. J., Vandongen, R., & Davidson, L. (1982). Epinephrine sulfation in the forearm: arteriovenous differences in free and conjugated catecholamines. *Life Sciences, 31*, 2513–2517.

Lake, C. R., Ziegler, M. G., & Kopin, I. J. (1976). Use of plasma norepinephrine for evaluation of sympathetic neuronal function in man. *Life Sciences, 18*, 1315–1326.

Landsberg, L., Greff, L, Gunn, S., & Young, J. B. (1980). Adrenergic mechanisms in the metabolic adaptation to fasting and feeding: Effects of phlorizin on diet-induced changes in sympathoadrenal activity in the rat. *Metabolism, 29*, 1128–1137.

Landsberg, L., Saville, M. E., & Young, J. B. (1984). The sympathoadrenal system and regulation of thermogenesis. *American Journal of Physiology, 247*, E181-E189.

Landsberg, L, & Young, J. B. (1983). Autonomic regulation of thermogenesis. In L. Girardier & M. J. Stock (Eds.), *Mammalian thermogenesis* (pp. 99–140). London, England: Chapman & Hall.

Landsberg, L., & Young, J. B. (1985a). Catecholamines and the adrenal medulla. In D. W. Foster & J. D. Wilson (Eds.), *Williams textbook of endocrinology* (7th ed, pp. 891–965). Philadelphia, PA: Saunders.

Landsberg, L., & Young, J. B. (1985b). The influence of diet on the sympathetic nervous system. In E. E. Muller, R. M. MacLeod, & L. A. Frohman (Eds.), *Neuroendocrine Perspectives* (pp. 191–218). Amsterdam, The Netherlands: Elsevier Science Publishers.

Landsberg, L., & Young, J. B. (1985c). Insulin-mediated glucose metabolism in the relationship between dietary intake and sympathetic nervous system activity. *International Journal of Obesity, 9*, 63–68.

Landsberg, L., & Young, J. B. (1986). Assessment of sympathetic nervous activity from measurements of noradrenaline turnover in rats. In M. H. Joseph, M. Fillenz, I. A. Macdonald, & C. A. Marsden (Eds.), *Monitoring neurotransmitter release during behaviour* (pp. 33–47). Chichester, England: Ellis Horwood Ltd.

Langley, L. L. (1973). *Homeostasis: Origins of the concept.* Stroudsburg, PA: Dowden, Hutchinson & Ross.

Lean, M. E. J., James, W. P. T., Jennings, G., & Trayhurn, P. (1986a). Brown adipose tissue uncoupling protein content in human infants, children, and adults. *Clinical Science, 71*, 291–297.

Lean, M. E. J., James, W. P. T., Jennings, G., & Trayhurn, P. (1986b). Brown adipose tissue in patients with phaeochromocytoma. *International Journal of Obesity, 10*, 219–227.

Leduc, J., (1961). Catecholamine production and release in exposure and acclimation to cold. *Acta Physiologica Scandinavica, 183* (Suppl), 1–101.

Lewis, G. P. (1975). Physiological mechanisms controlling secretory activity of adrenal medulla. In R. O. Greep, E. B. Astwood, H. Blaschko, G. Sayers, G. Smith, & S. R. Geiger (Eds.), *Handbook of physiology* (pp. 309–319). Baltimore, MD: Waverly Press.

Loggie, J. M. H., & Van Maanen, E. F. (1972). The autonomic nervous system and some aspects of the use of autonomic drugs in children. *Journal of Pediatrics, 81*(2), 205–216.

Maickel, R., Susman, H., Yamada, K., & Brodie, B. (1963). Control of adipose tissue lipase activity by the sympathetic nervous system. *Life Sciences, 3*, 210–214.

Maickel, R. P., Matussek, N., Stern, D. N., & Brodie, B. B. (1967). The sympathetic nervous system as a homeostatic mechanism. I. Absolute need for sympathetic nervous function in body temperature maintenance of cold-exposed rats. *Journal of Pharmacology and Experimental Therapeutics, 157*, 103–110.

Marcus, C., Karpe, B., Bolme, P., Sonnenfeld, T., & Arner, P. (1987). Changes in catecholamine-induced lipolysis in isolated human fat cells during the first year of life. *Journal of Clinical Investigation, 79*, 1812–1818.

Mason, J. W., Hartley, L. H., Kotchen, T. A., Mougey, E. H., Ricketts, P. T., & Jones, L. R. G. (1973). Plasma cortisol and norepinephrine responses in anticipation of muscular exercise. *Psychosomatic Medicine, 35*, 406–414.

Moss, A. J., & Wynar, B. (1970). Tachycardia in house officers presenting cases at grand rounds. *Annals of Internal Medicine, 72*, 255–256.

Oliver, J. A., Pinto, J., Sciacca, R. R., & Cannon, P. J. (1980). Increased renal secretion of norepinephrine and prostaglandin E_2 during sodium depletion in the dog. *Journal of Clinical Investigation*, 66, 748–756.

Pomeranz, B. H., Birtch, A. G., & Barger, A. C. (1968). Neural control of intrarenal blood flow. *American Journal of Physiology, 215*, 1067–1081.

Rappaport, E. B., Young, J. B., & Landsberg, L. (1982). Effects of 2-deoxy-D-glucose on the cardiac sympathetic nerves and the adrenal medulla in the rat: Further evidence for a dissociation of sympathetic nervous system and adrenal medullary responses. *Endocrinology, 110*, 650–656.

Raven, P. B., Niki, I., Dahms, T. E., & Horvath, S. M. (1970). Compensatory cardiovascular responses during an environmental cold stress, 5°C. *Journal of Applied Physiology, 19*, 417–421.

Robin, E. D. (1979). *Claude Bernard and the internal environment.* New York: Marcel Dekker.

Seitz, H. J., Krone, W., Wilke, W., & Tarnowski, W. (1981). Rapid raise in plasma glucagon induced by acute cold exposure in man and rat. *Pflugers Archive, 389*, 115–120.

Silva, P., Landsberg, L., & Besarab, A. (1979). Excretion and metabolism of catecholamines by the isolated perfused rat kidney. *Journal of Clinical Investigation, 64*, 850–857.

Silverberg, A. B., Shah, S. D., Haymond, M. W., & Cryer, P. E. (1978). Norepinephrine: hormone and neurotransmitter in man. *American Journal of Physiology, 234*, E252-E256.

Sjostrom, L., Schutz, Y., Gudinchet, F., Hegnell, L., Pittet, P. G., & Jequier, E. (1983). Epinephrine sensitivity with respect to metabolic rate and other variables in women. *American Journal of Physiology, 245*, E431–E442.

Taggart, P., Carruthers, M., & Somerville, W. (1973). Electrocardiogram, plasma catecholamines and lipids, and their modification by oxprenolol when speaking before an audience. *Lancet, 1*, 341–346.

Taggart, P., Hedworth-Whitty, R., Carruthers, M., & Gordon, P. D. (1976). Observations on electrocardiogram and plasma catecholamines during dental procedures: The forgotten vagus. *British Medical Journal, 2*, 787–789.

Wallin, B. G., Sundlof, G., Eriksson, B-M., Dominiak, P., Grobecker, H., & Lindblad, L. E. (1981). Plasma noradrenaline correlates to sympathetic muscle nerve activity in normotensive man. *Acta Physiologica Scandinavica, 111*, 69–73.

Webb-Peploe, M. M., & Shepard, J. T. (1975). Responses of the superficial limb veins of the dog to changes in temperature. *Circulation Research, 22*, 737–746.

Williams, M., Young, J. B., Rosa, R. M., Gunn, S., Epstein, F. H., & Landsberg, L. (1986). Effects of protein ingestion on urinary dopamine excretion: evidence for the functional importance of renal decarboxylation of circulating 3, 4-dihydroxyphenylalanine (DOPA) in man. *Journal of Clinical Investigation, 78*, 1687–1693.

Young, J. B., Fish, S., & Landsberg, L. (1983). Sympathetic nervous system and adrenal medullar responses to ischemic injury in mice. *American Journal of Physiology, 245,* E67–E73.

Young, J. B., & Landsberg, L. (1977). Suppression of sympathetic nervous system during fasting. *Science, 196,* 1473–1475.

Young, J. B., & Landsberg, L. (1979a). Sympathoadrenal activity in fasting pregnant rats: dissociation of adrenal medullary and sympathetic nervous system responses. *Journal of Clinical Investigation, 64,* 109–116.

Young, J. B., & Landsberg, L. (1979b). Effect of diet and cold exposure on norepinephrine turnover in pancreas and liver. *American Journal of Physiology, 236,* E524-E533.

Young, J. B., & Landsberg, L. (1980). Impaired suppression of sympathetic activity during fasting in the gold thioglucose-treated mouse. *Journal of Clinical Investigation, 65,* 1086–1094.

Young, J. B., & Landsberg, L. (1981). Effect of concomitant fasting and cold exposure on sympathoadrenal activity in rats. *American Journal of Physiology, 240,* E314-E319.

Young, J. B., Rosa, R. M., & Landsberg, L. (1984). Dissociation of sympathetic nervous system and adrenal medullary responses. *American Journal of Physiology, 247,* E34–E40.

Young, J. B., Saville, M. E., Rothwell, N. J., Stock, M. J., & Landsberg, L. (1982). Effect of diet and cold exposure on norepinephrine turnover in brown adipose tissue in the rat. *Journal of Clinical Investigation, 69,* 1061–1071.

4

Neuropeptides and Their Receptors as the Biochemicals of Emotion

Joanna M. Hill
National Institute of Mental Health

One of the most significant events in modern neurobiology was the discovery by Ernst and Berta Sharrer (1940) that neurons of the hypothalamus synthesize hormones. This discovery was closely followed by the realization that several additional hypothalamic hormones, released into the capillary bed of the hypophyseal stalk, were transported to the anterior pituitary where they regulated anterior pituitary function. The field of neuroendocrinology developed from these discoveries and contributed, among other things, two new and important ideas to biology. First, the detection of hormone-secreting cells in the brain helped to remove the distinction between neurons and endocrine cells and led to a better understanding of the evolutionary development of the endocrine and nervous systems. Second, the feedback regulatory mechanisms in the neuroendocrine system, whereby the secretion of hypothalamic-releasing factors is regulated by the levels of the target organ secretions, replaced the predominant hierarchical views of physiological function with an understanding of the interdependence, and multidirectional communications between systems of the body. The pituitary was no longer the master gland, but a link in the complex mechanism of homeostasis.

Recent progress in neuroscience research has resulted in the formation of some new ideas that may have an equal impact on the future understanding of neurobiology. This chapter reviews some of these new ideas and shows how they lead to the hypothesis that neuropeptides and their receptors not only form the biochemical framework for a communication network in the emotion-mediating regions of the brain but also, perhaps, the framework for a communication system throughout the body.

PARASYNAPTIC INFORMATION TRANSMISSION

Recent investigations have lead to the hypothesis that: in addition to classical synaptic transmission, interneuronal communication may occur by the diffusion of information substances[1] through the extracellular fluid of the brain to act upon receptors on noncontiguous neurons.

F. O. Schmitt (1984) called this phenomenon "parasynaptic transmission" because it exists in parallel with synapse-linked circuitry. He has pointed out that, in addition to the selectivity of the synaptic system, the parasynaptic system has much versatility and plasticity and is influenced by the multitude of informational substances in the ambient extracellular fluid.

R. Nieuwenhuys (1985) has proposed a similar nonsynaptic "paracrine mode of interneuronal communication" whereby informational substances released into the extracellular fluid by thin, unmyelinated fibers coursing through the core of the brain can influence numerous adjacent neurons.

M. Herkenham (1987; Herkenham & McLean, 1986) has likewise proposed the "action at a distance" of neuroactive substances in the brain to explain the mismatch of information substances and their receptors in the brain. In an extensive review, Herkenham and his colleagues report that a correspondence in the localization of an informational substance in perikarya and terminals of neurons and the receptors for that informational substance is the exception rather than the rule. In some cases, "the patterns are not merely dissimilar but virtually complementary" (p. 137).

The study of neuroanatomy has been focused on attempting to understand the relationships between the cytoarchitecturally different regions of the brain by determining the input–output patterns of distinct cell groups. By these means an understanding of the relationships and functions of brain regions can be gained. Recent tract-tracing methods have resulted in a much expanded knowledgeof the pathways of nerve fibers in the brain and have revealed amazinglycomplex synaptic connections of the brain. On top of this already complex synaptic communication system is overlaid the complex parasynaptic communication system suggested here. Brain regions not connected by fiber pathways can communicate by the diffusion of informational substances through the extracellular spaces separating them.

PEPTIDES AS MESSAGES IN THE BRAIN AND BODY

Numerous peptides and their receptors are present throughout the brain where they modulate neuronal function and behavior.

[1]The use of the term *informational substance* in this chapter stems from the suggestion by Schmitt (1984) that this term be used for the regulators of the central nervous system including neurotransmitters, hormones, and other neuroactive substances found in the brain.

That peptide hormones function as messages between cells throughout the body has been well documented. The pituitary, pancreatic, and intestinal hormones are peptides and are transported from their point of secretion to act on the receptors of their target cells via the extracellular fluid of the circulatory system. That peptides are present in the brain was recognized in the 1950s when oxytocin and vasopressin, the hypothalamic hormones discovered by the Sharrers (1940), as previously discussed, were found to be nonapeptides (Pierce & Vigneaud, 1950; Popenoe & Vigneaud, 1954). In the early 1970s it was learned that the many other hypothalamic hormones, acting as releasing factors, was also peptides. However, only after the demonstration that potently neuroactive neuropeptides, such as somatostatin (Vale et al., 1975), and thyrotropin-releasing hormone (Morley, 1979), were widely distributed throughout the brain, that opiate peptides (Hughes et al., 1975) and their receptors (Pert & Snyder, 1973) were present in the brain and the discovery that the neuroactive compounds neurotensin and substance P were neuropeptides (Carraway & Leeman, 1973; Brazeau et al., 1973) was it fully recognized that neuropeptides composed an important, and possibly the largest, class of informational substance in the brain.

At this writing, about 50 peptides have been found in the brain (Table 4.1); however, this number represents only about one quarter of the total number predicted (Snyder, 1980; Sternberger, 1980).

Peptides have a number of characteristics which make them particularly suitable as informational substances in the brain (Schmitt, 1984). They are biologically active at extremely low concentrations, can be synthesized by the cleavage of a larger precursor molecule, they often coexist with classical neurotransmitters, can be transported in extracellular fluids some distance before being degraded, and can act as intercellular signals at synapses, or parasynaptically as described earlier.

NEUROPEPTIDE DISTRIBUTION IN THE BRAIN

In an extensive review of the chemoarchitecture of the brain, Nieuwenhuys (1985) has shown that: the set of brain regions enriched with information substances, primarily neuropeptides, overlaps extensively with the limbic system.

This colocalization of neuropeptides with the limbic regions of the brain suggests that they may play an important role in limbic functions; namely, the modulation of affective and motivational behavior.

NEUROPEPTIDE RECEPTOR DISTRIBUTION IN THE BRAIN

Because neuropeptide release points can be some distance from sites of synthesis, and neuropeptides may diffuse from the site of release to receptors on

TABLE 4.1
Neuropeptides

Adrenocorticotropic hormone	Melatonin
Angiotensin I	(Met)enkephalin
Angiotensin II	Motilin
Angiotensin III	Nerve growth factor
Bombesin	Neurohypophysial hormone
Bradykinin	Neuropeptide Y
Calcitonin	Neurophysin
Calcitonin gene-related peptide	Neurotensin
Carnosine	Oxytocin
Cholecystokinin	Pancreatic polypeptides
Corticotropic-releasing factor	Physalaemin
Ependymin (β and γ)	Pituitary peptides
β-Endorphin	Proctolin
Gastrin	Prolactin
Gastrointestinal polypeptide	Secretin
Glucagon	Somatostatin
Gonadotropin–releasing hormone	Substance K
Growth hormone	Substance P
Hypothalamic–releasing hormone	Thyroid hormone
Insulin	Thyroid–stimulating hormone
Insulin–like growth factor I	Thyrotropin–releasing hormone
Insulin–like growth factor II	Transferrin
Interleukin I	Arginine vasopressin
(Leu)enkephalin	Lysine vasopressin
Luteinizing hormone	Vasoactive intestinal polypeptide
Luteinizing hormone-releasing factor	Vasotocin
Melanocyte–stimulating hormone (α and β)	
Melanocyte–stimulating hormone-releasing hormone	

noncontinguous neurons, the specificity of neuropeptide function is determined largely by the localization and densities of receptors.

The development of autoradiographic techniques in the mid-1970s led to the determination of the distribution patterns of receptors for neuropeptides throughout the brain. Although each type of receptor was found to have a characteristic distribution pattern, limbic structures, especially the amygdala and hippocampus, seemed to have receptors for every neuropeptide studied (Pert et al., 1985).

A more or less complete description of the distribution patterns of the receptors for 22 neuropeptides has been accomplished and we have analyzed these recptor patterns to determine which brain regions are typically enriched with neuropeptide receptors and if the enriched areas are limbic and associated regions (Hill, Zipser, & Pert, 1988).

Twenty-three brain regions were found to be enriched (Table 4.2, i.e., having 55% or more of the 22 peptides). Figure 4.1 illustrates the receptor distribution

TABLE 4.2
Peptide Receptor Rich Brain Regions

	AII	AVP	BN	CT	CGRP	CCK	CRF	INS	IGF-I	IGF-II	IL-1	NGF	NPY	NT	OP	OT	SS	SK	SP	TRH	TF	VIP	%
1. Amygdala	+	+	+	+	+	+	+	+	+	+	+	0	+	+	+	+	+	+	+	+	+	+	95
2. Dentate gyrus	+	+	+	0	+	+	+	+	+	+	+	+	+	+	+	0	+	+	+	+	+	+	91
3. Hippocampus proper	+	+	+	0	0	+	+	+	+	+	+	+	+	+	+	0	+	+	+	+	+	+	86
4. Cerebral cortex	+	+	+	0	+	+	+	+	+	+	+	0	+	+	+	0	+	+	+	+	+	+	86
5. Caudate putamen	0	+	+	+	+	+	+	+	+	+	+	0	+	+	+	0	+	+	+	0	+	+	82
6. Olfactory bulb	+	+	+	?	?	+	+	+	+	+	+	?	?	+	+	?	+	+	+	+	+	+	77
7. Septum	+	+	0	+	0	+	+	+	0	0	+	+	+	+	+	+	+	+	+	+	+	0	77
8. Central grey	+	0	+	+	+	+	+	+	0	0	+	0	+	+	+	0	+	+	+	+	+	+	77
9. Paraventricular nucleus	+	+	+	+	0	0	+	+	+	+	0	0	+	0	0	+	+	+	+	+	+	+	73
10. Nucleus accumbens	0	+	+	+	+	+	+	+	+	0	+	0	0	+	+	0	0	0	+	+	+	+	68
11. Nuclei of stria terminalis/ stria terminalis	0	+	+	+	0	+	+	+	+	0	0	0	+	+	+	+	+	0	0	+	+	+	68
12. Subiculum	+	+	+	0	0	+	+	+	0	+	+	0	0	+	+	+	0	0	+	+	+	+	68
13. Superior colliculus, superficial grey	+	0	+	0	+	+	+	+	+	0	+	0	0	+	+	0	+	0	+	+	+	+	68
14. Interpeduncular nucleus	+	0	+	+	0	+	+	+	+	0	0	+	0	0	+	0	+	+	+	+	+	+	68
15. Substantia gelatinosa	+	0	+	0	0	?	+	+	+	+	?	+	+	+	+	0	+	+	+	+	?	+	68
16. Entorhinal cortex	0	+	0	0	+	+	+	+	+	+	+	0	0	0	+	0	+	0	+	+	+	+	64
17. Nucleus of the solitary tract	+	+	+	+	+	+	+	0	0	0	0	0	0	+	+	0	+	+	+	+	0	+	64
18. Olfactory tubercle	0	0	+	0	+	+	+	+	0	0	0	0	+	+	0	+	+	0	+	+	+	+	59
19. Cingulate cortex	0	0	+	0	0	+	+	+	0	+	+	0	0	+	+	0	+	0	+	+	+	+	59
20. Cerebellar cortex, molecular layer	+	+	0	0	+	0	+	+	+	+	+	0	+	+	0	0	0	0	0	+	+	+	59
21. Medial preoptic area	+	0	+	+	0	+	0	+	0	0	+	0	0	+	0	0	+	0	+	+	+	+	55
22. Medial habenula	+	0	0	0	+	0	+	0	0	+	+	0	0	+	+	0	+	0	+	+	+	+	55
23. Locus coeruleus	+	0	+	+	+	+	0	0	0	+	0	0	0	+	+	0	+	0	+	0	+	+	55

Peptide receptor rich regions of the brain: +, receptor present; o, few or no receptors; ?, unreported; AII, angiotensin II; AVP, arginine–vasopressin; BN, Bombesin; CT, calcitonin; CGRP, calcitonin gene-related peptide; CCK, cholecystokinin; CRF, corticotropin releasing factor; INS, insulin; 1GF–I, insuline-like growth factor–I; 1GF–II, insulin-like growth factor II: IL–1, interleukin–I; NGF, nerve growth factor; NPY, neuropeptide Y; NT, neurotensin; OP, opiates; OT, oxytocin; SS, somatostatin; SK, substance K; SP, substance P; TRH, thyrotropin-releasing hormone; Tf, transferrin; VIP, vasoactive intestinal peptide. Revised from Hill et al. (1988).

patterns for seven of the neuropeptides studied, on five different brain sections ranging from rostral forebrain, to medulla or spinal cord. The receptor patterns for classical neuropeptides (opiates, substance P, and neurotensin), hormones (insulin, somatostatin, and cholecystokinin, and a growth factor (transferrin) are represented. The receptor-rich regions of the brain were found to be widespread and to encompass diverse brain structures involved in diverse functions. In addition, we determined that: the neuropeptide receptor-enriched areas of the brain overlap extensively with limbic and associated regions.

The neuropeptide receptor-rich regions of the brain are depicted in Fig. 4.1, and 4.2 illustrates their relation to limbic structures.

Although there is no true consensus as to the composition of the limbic system, the classical limbic regions (Fig. 4.2b) usually consist of the structures of Papez (1937) circuit, (the hypothalamus, anterior thalamic nucleus, cingulate gyrus, and hippocampus), and those regions included by MacLean (1952), the amygdala and many cortical and subcortical regions having reciprocal connections with the hypothalamus. The receptor-rich regions of the brain overlapping with these classical limbic areas and others, such as the striatum, parts of which have recently been found to have reciprocal hypothalamic connections (Gerfen, 1984; Kelly, Domesick, & Nauta, 1982), appear in black in Fig. 4.2b (the cortex appearing in Fig. 4.2b represents the limbic cortex, i.e., the basal fronto–temporal region having reciprocal connections with the amygdala and/or hypothalamus). Nauta and Domesick (1982) have expanded the concept of the limbic system by including a number of strongly interconnected mesencephalic structures. Together with the forebrain limbic structures, these form a functional system the "limbic system–midbrain circuit." The receptor-rich regions of the brain included in this circuit appear in dark gray in Fig. 4.2b. The limbic system is further characterized by the identification of a limbic system specific antigen,a surface marker, recently isolated through monoclonal antibodies and postulated to play a role in the system's assembly (Levitt, 1984). This antigen is expressed by most of the limbic and associated regions appearing in black and grey in Fig. 4.2b, and three other brain regions, the substantia gelatinosa, the superficial layer of the superior colliculus, and the molecular layer of the cerebellar cortex (Fig. 4.2b, pale grey) previously not considered to be limbic–associated areas. However, Haines and Dietrichs (1987) have reported reciprocal connections between the cerebellum and the hypothalamus. Also, the superior colliculus has been shown to receive synaptic input from the cingulate cortex (Domesick, 1969; Siegel, Troiano, & Royce, 1973).

Our demonstration that neuropeptide receptor-enriched regions of the brain overlap with the limbic and associated regions supports the concept of neuropeptides as the biochemicals of emotion. In addition, they suggest that neuropeptide receptor-rich regions of the brain form nodes in an emotion mediating network of the brain.

THE LIMBIC SYSTEM CONCEPT

The concept of the limbic system was originally based on the reciprocal connectivity of regions through neuronal pathways. Modern track-tracing methods have greatly expanded the number of brain regions included in the "limbic system," by this definition. At the same time, however, these methods have demonstrated that the interconnections among the various components of the original Papez circuit of emotions may not be the major connections of these structures. This has resulted in the opinion, by some, that the term *limbic system* should be abolished, that Papez circuit is of historical interest only (Brodal, 1981), and that the concept of the limbic system has perhaps outlived its usefulness (Heimer, 1983).

These criticisms, however valid, do not solve the problem of understanding the relation of emotion to brain structures. Certain brain regions are involved in the subjective feeling and expression of emotions. The hypothalamus, through its connections with the brain stem, regulates the expression of emotion. Therefore, brain regions with reciprocal hypothalamic connects are in a position to modify emotional expression. Ablation and stimulation experiments have identified other brain regions, for example, the amygdala, cingulate gyrus, frontal cortex, septum/hippocampus, and locus coeruleus, which are involved somehow in the emotionality of the organism. Therefore, these regions and those to which they are connected can modulate emotion.

The combination of recent developments and new ideas outlined in this chapter can, perhaps, be put together to create a new view of the regulation of emotion.

Levitts' (1984) discovery of a limbic system specific antigen provides a molecular basis for linking the limbic regions. Similarly, Nieuwenhuys' (1985) finding that the "neuromediator-rich" regions of the brain constitute a "readily recognizable entity" that coincides largely with the limbic system, including the midbrain structures outlined by Nauta and Domesick (1982), suggests that limbic regions share both molecular and biochemical characteristics that bring them together as an entity. Our study of the peptide receptor-rich regions of the brain (Hill et al., submitted) both complements and extends the concept that the regions share molecular and biochemical features. The neuropeptide receptor-rich regions of the brain form a recognizable entity which encompasses regions brought together originally on an anatomical basis and later on by molecular/biochemical similarities.

Although there is a mismatch between the sites of a neuropeptides release and the localization of its receptors (Herkenham, 1987; Herkenham & McLean, 1986), both the receptors, as we have shown (Hill et al., 1988) and the peptides, as shown by Nieuwenhuys (1985) are enriched in the limbic regions of the brain.

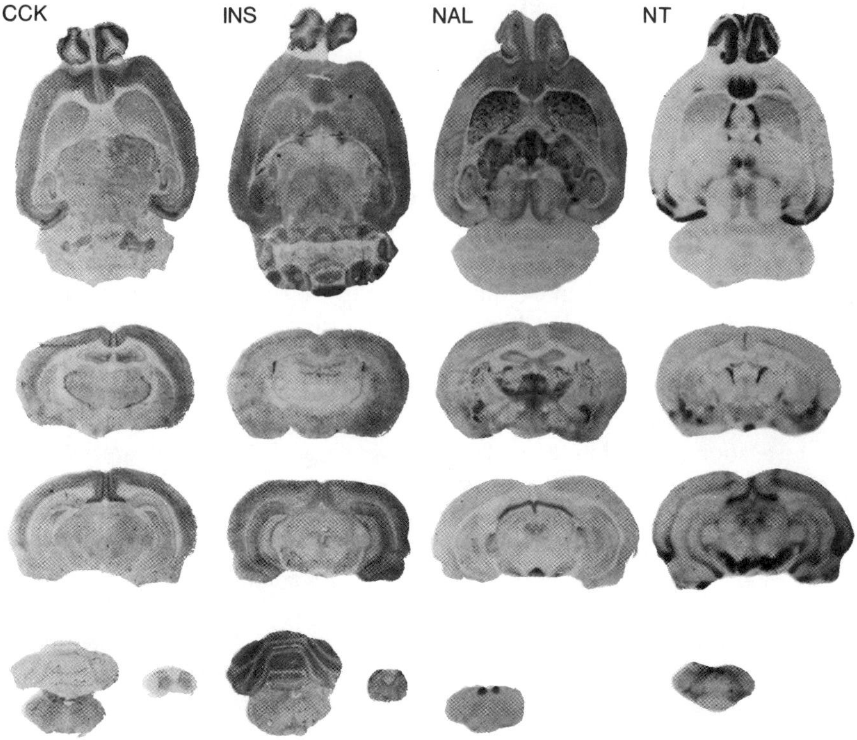

(a)

FIG. 4.1. Film (a. b.) autoradiographs illustrating the receptor distribution patterns of seven different neuropeptides in the horizontal plane, and coronal view at the level of the thalamus and amygdala, at the level of the superior colliculus and hippocampus, at the level of the cerebellum and medulla, and at the level of the spinal cord. From Hill et al. (1988).

Abbreviations: AMY, amygdala; CCK, cholecystokinin; CC, mol, cerebellar cortex, molecular layer; CG, central grey; CIC, cingulate cortex; CPu, caudate putamen; CTX, cortex; DG, dentate gyrus; H, hippocampus; INS, insulin; M. Hab, medial habenula; NAL, naloxone; NT, neurotensin; OB, olfactory bulb; PaN, paraventricular nucleus; S, septum; SC, superior colliculus; SG, substantia gelatinosa; Sol, nucleus solitarius; SON, supraoptic nucleus; SP, substance P; Su, subiculum; TF, transferrin; VIP, vasoactive intestinal peptide; A, film autoradiographs for CCK, INS, NAL and NT,B. film autoradiographs for SP, TF, VIP and line drawings with brain regions labeled. Tissue was prepared as described (Herkenham & Pert, 1982) and serial brain sections radiolabeled according to the following procedures: CCK (Guadreau et al., 1983), INS (Hill et al., 1986), NAL (Herkenham & Pert, 1982), NT (Quirion et al., 1982), TF (Hill et al., 1985), VIP (Wiedermann et al., 1987).

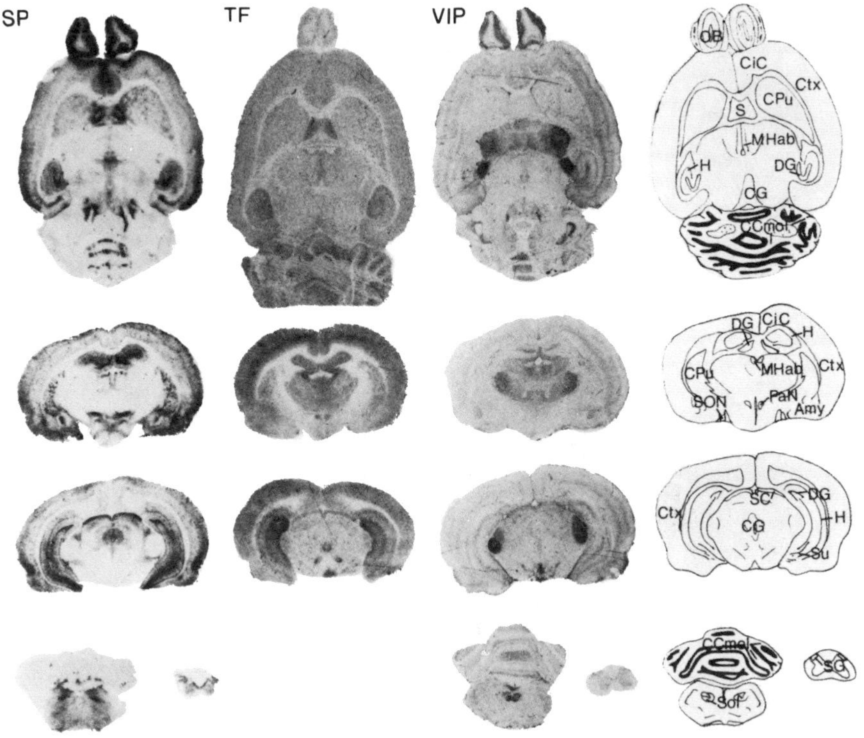

(b)

The neuropeptide-rich limbic regions of the brain can communicate with the neuropeptide receptor-rich limbic regions of the brain not only through a multitude of reciprocal synaptic pathways, but also through the extensive and versatile parasynaptic system. There are potentially 200 neuropeptides and their receptors concentrated in the limbic and associated structures of the brain; peptides that are potent at extremely low concentrations and can diffuse for considerable time and distance before being degraded.

Therefore, what the "limbic system" lacks in synaptic communication through strong anatomical connections between its various components, perhaps is made up for by a potentially extensive parasynaptic communication.

This collection of brain regions may not function as a system in the same way as a neuronal circuit as originally invisioned by Papez (1937) or the documented circuits of the brain that today are referred to as systems. However, a function as complex as the modulation or emotion, requiring the integration and coordi-

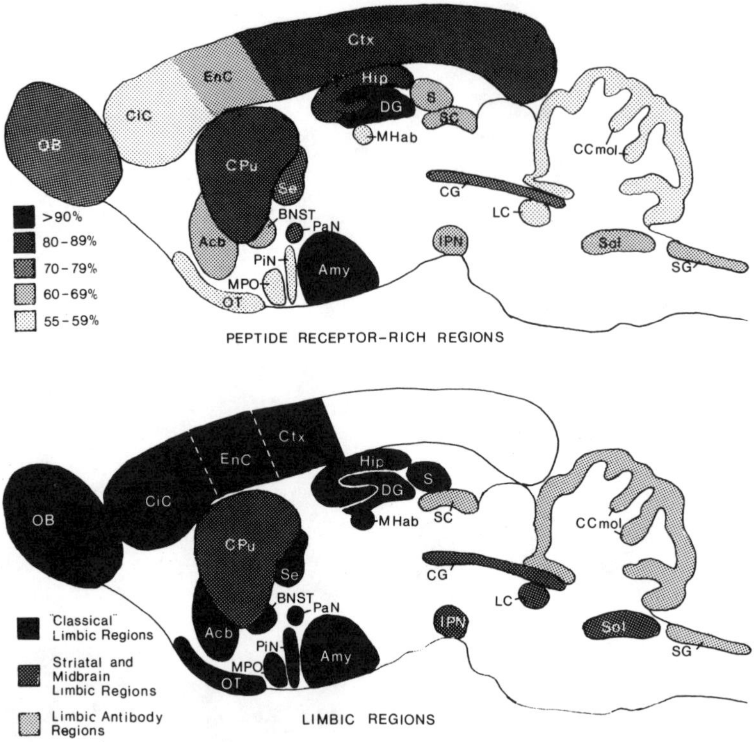

FIG. 4.2. Line drawings illustrating the peptide receptor–rich regions of the brain (upper drawing) and the limbic regions of the brain (lower drawing) in which peptide receptors are enriched. Shades of grey in upper drawing correspond to the percentage of the 22 different peptide receptors found in each brain region. See Table 4.2. Shades of grey in lower drawing depict which peptide receptor–rich brain regions are considered classical limbic regions, (Papez, 1937; MacLean, 1952) striatal (Gerfen, 1984; Kelly et al., 1982) and midbrain limbic regions (Nauta & Domesick, 1982) and limbic antibody regions (Levitt, 1984) see text for further discussion. Revised from Hill et al. (1988).

Abbreviations: Acb, nucleus accumbens; Amy, amygdala; BNST, bed nucleus of the stria terminalis; CC mol, cerebellar cortex, molecular layer; CG, central grey; CiC, cingulate cortex; CPu, caudate putamen; Ctx, cortex; DG, denate gyrus; En C, entorihinal cortex; Hip, hippocampus; IPN, interpeduncular nucleus; LC, locus, coeruleus; M Hab, medial habenula; MPD, medial preoptic area; OB, olfactory bulb, OT, olfactory tubercle; PaN paraventricular nucleus; PiN, periventricular nucleus; S, subiculum; SC, superior colliculus; Se, septum; SG, substantia gelatinosa; Sol, nucleus solitarius.

nation of the perceptions of both the internal and external milieu perhaps requires much of the brain and includes regions which overlap with many other systems of the brain.

NEUROPEPTIDE AND NEUROPEPTIDE RECEPTOR-ENRICHED REGIONS OF THE BODY AND THEIR RELATION TO EMOTION

Most of the peptides and their receptors listed in Table 4.1, were originally discovered in other parts of the body and only later found to be present in the brain. The opposite is also true. Neuropeptides and neuropeptide receptors, such as the opiates, originally found in the brain have been found widely distributed throughout the body. The discovery that the brain and body utilize a common set of peptides and their receptors has important implications in understanding the relation between emotion and health. Shared peptides and peptide receptors may form a molecular/biochemical framework for a bidirectional communication network between brain and body (Pert, Ruff, Weber, & Henkenham, 1985).

Peptides synthesized throughout the body and entering the brain through the circumventricular organs, crossing the blood–brain barrier, or being brought in by migrating macrophages can gain access to brain receptors. Thus, informational substances in the extracellular fluid reaching limbic receptors from any part of the brain or body, can potentially modify emotions.

Further, if the neuropeptide receptor rich regions of the brain form nodes in an emotion mediating network of the brain, perhaps the neuropeptide receptor rich regions of the body can also be considered nodes in this communication network (Hill et al., 1988).

ACKNOWLEDGMENTS

I gratefully acknowledge the excellent technical assistance of Ms. Nicole Jelesoff and Ms. Sabine Jean-Paul. I also thank Mrs. Mary Flanagan Cyr and Ms. Yolanda Edwards for their careful preparation of this manuscript.

REFERENCES

Brazeau, P., Vale, W., Burgus, R., Ling, N., Butcher, M., Rivier, J., & Guillemin, R. (1973). Hypothalamic polypeptide that inhibits the secretion of immunoreactive pituitary growth hormone. *Science, 179*, 77–79.

Brodal, A. (1981). *Neurological anatomy in relation to clinical medicine* (3rd ed.). New York: Oxford University Press.

Carraway, R., & Leeman, S. E. (1973). The isolation of a new hypothalamic peptide, neurotensin, from the bovine hypothalami. *Journal of Biological Chemistry, 248*,

Domesick, V. B. (1969). Projections from the cingulate cortex in the rat. *Brain Research, 12*, 296–320.
Guadreau, P., Quirion, R., St-Pierre, S., & Pert, C. B. (1983). Characterization and visualization of cholecystokinin receptors in rat brain using (^{3}H) pentagastrin. *Peptides, 4*, 755–762.
Gerfen, C. R. (1984). The neostriatalmosaic: compartmentalization of corticostriatal input and striatonigral output systems. *Nature, 311*, 461–464.
Haines, P. E., & Dietrichs, E. (1987). On the organization of interconnections between the cerebellum and hypothalamus. In J. S. King (Ed.), *New concepts in cerebellar neurobiology* (pp. 113–149). New York: Alan R. Liss.
Heimer, L. (1983). *The human brain and spinal cord. The functional neuroanatomy and dissection guide.* New York: Springer-Verlag.
Herkenham, M. (1987). Mismatches between neurotransmitter and receptor localizations in brain. Observations and implications. *Neuroscience, 23*, 1–38.
Herkenham, M., & McLean, S. (1986). Mismatches between receptor and transmitter localizations in the brain, observations and implications. In C. Boast, E. W. Snowhill, & C. A. Altar (Eds.), *Quantitative receptor autoradiography* (pp. 137–171). New York: Alan R. Liss.
Herkenham, M., & Pert, C. B. (1982). Light microscopic localization of brain opiate receptors: A general autoradiographic method which preserve tissue quality. *Journal of Neuroscience, 24*, 1129–1149.
Hill, J. M., Lesniak, M. A., Pert, C. B., & Roth, J. (1986). Autoradiographic localization of insulin receptors in rat brain: prominence in olfactory and limbic areas. *Neuroscience, 17*, 1127–1138.
Hill, J. M., Ruff, M. R., Weber, R. J., & Pert, C. B. (1985). Transferrin receptors in rat brain: neuropeptide-like pattern and relationship to iron distribution. *Proceedings of the National Academy of Science USA, 82*, 4553–4557.
Hill, J. M., Zipser, B., & Pert, C. B. (1988). *Neuropeptide receptors enriched in limbic and associated structures.* Manuscript submitted for publication.
Hughes, J., Smith, T. W., Koslerlitz, H. W., Fathergill, L. A., Morgan, B. A., & Morris, H. R. (1975). Identification of two related pentapeptides from brain with potent agonist activity. *Nature, 258*, 577–580.
Kelly, A. E., Domesick, V. B., & Nauta, W. J. H. (1982). The amygdalostriatal projections in the rat. An anatomical study by anterograde and retrograde tracing methods. *Neuroscience, 1*, 615–630.
Levitt, P. (1984). A monoclonal antibody to limbic system neurons. *Science, 223*, 299–301.
MacLean, P. D. (1952). Some psychiatric implications of physiological studies on frontotemporal portion of limbic system (visceral brain). *EEG and Clinical Neurophysiology Journal, 4*, 407–418.
Morley, J. E (1979). Extrahypothalamic thyrotropin releasing hormone (TRH): Its distribution and its functions. *Life Science, 25*, 1539–1550.
Nauta, W. J. H., & Domesick, V. B. (1982). Neural associations of the limbic system. In A. L. Beckman (Ed.), *The neurological basis of behavior* (pp. 175–206). New York: Spectrum.
Nieuwenhuys, R. (1985). *Chemoarchitecture of the brain.* New York: Springer-Verlag.
Papez, J. W. (1937). A proposed mechanism of emotion. *Archives of Neurology of*

Psychiatry, 38, 725–743.

Pert, C. B., Ruff, M. R., Weber, R. J., & Herkenham, M. (1985). Neuropeptides and their receptors: A psychosomatic network. *Journal of Immunology, 135,* 820s–826s.

Pert, C. B., & Snyder, S. H. (1973). Opiate receptor: Demonstration in nervous tissue. *Science, 179,* 1011–1014.

Pierce, J. G., & du Vigneaud, V. (1950). Preliminary studies on amino acid content of a high protein preparation of the oxytoxic hormone of posterior lobe of the pituitary gland. *Journal of Biological Chemistry, 182,* 359–366.

Popenoe, N. A., & du Vigneaud, V. (1954). A partial sequence of amino acid in performic acid-oxidized vasopressin. *Journal of Biological Chemistry, 202,* 353–360.

Quirion, R., Guadreau, P., St.-Pierre, S., Rioux, F., & Pert, C. B. (1982). Autoradiographic distribution of (^{3}H) neurotensin receptors in rat brain; visualization by tritium sensitive film. *Peptides, 3,* 757–763.

Schmitt, F. O. (1984). Molecular regulators of brain function: A new view. *Neuroscience, 13,* 991–1001.

Sharrer, E., & Sharrer, B. (1940). Secretory cells within the hypothalamus. *Research Publications Association for Research in Nervous and Mental Disease, 20,* 170–194.

Siegel, A., Troiano, R., & Royce, A. (1973). Differential projections of the anterior and posterior cingulate gyrus to the thalamus in the cat. *Experimental Neurology, 38,* 192–201.

Snyder, S. H. (1980). Brain peptides as neurotransmitters. *Science, 209,* 976–983.

Sternberger, L. A. (1980). What is brain? An immunocytochemical neuroendocrine approach. *Acta Histochemica et. Cytochemica, 13,* 66–70.

Vale, W., Brazeau, P., Rivier, C., Brown, M., Bass, B., Rivier, J., Burgus, R., Ling, N., & Guillemin, R. (1975). Somatostatin. *Recent Progress in Hormone Research, 34,* 365–397.

Wiedermann, C. J., Sertl, K., Zipser, B., Hill, J. M., & Pert, C. B. (1987). Vasoactive intestinal peptide receptors in rat spleen and brain: A shared communication network. *Peptides, 9,* (Suppl. 1), 21–28.

5

Analysis of Stress Susceptibility Using the Maudsley Reactive and Non-Reactive Strains

David A. Blizard
Bowman Gray School of Medicine of Wake Forest University

Coping with the uncertainty generated by social situations evokes wide differences in behavioral and physiological response patterns among primate species including man (see Kagan et al. and Levine & Wiener, this volume). There is great interest in the central nervous system (CNS) mechanisms underlying these differences: The individual variations in psychophysiological response emerge early in ontogeny, and psychologists have been willing to consider the possibility that they are genetically mediated because their early appearance is presumed less likely to be dependent on environmental influences. Genetic influences can be investigated in man but the rich variety of genetic models that exist in rodent species provide an excellent resource in this field. These models offer the usual conveniences of investigation with small, laboratory-reared animals and permit a more detailed and rigorous analysis of underlying physiological and biochemical mechanisms.

THE MAUDSLEY MODEL

A variety of rodent genetic models exist for exploration of coping with the uncertainty generated by both social and other environmental stimuli (Adams & Blizard, 1987; Blizard & Fulker, 1981). I discuss research involving use of the Maudsley rat strains that were selected for differences in open-field defecation (OFD) in the United Kingdom by Peter Broadhurst in the late 1950s and early 1960s (Broadhurst, 1960, 1962). They were developed to provide an animal model of the human personality dimension of emotionality (Eysenck, 1967) or, as more specifically enunciated by Broadhurst (1956) to investigate "the part played by individual differences in emotional responses in the development of particular patterns of behavior." (p. 4). The term *development* in the preceding usage does not refer to ontogeny but rather to the sequential elaboration of particular patterns of behavior in a specific test situation.

The Validity of Open-Field Defecation. An open field consists of well-illuminated, open space circumscribed by square or circular walls and is assumed to be aversive for the photo- and agerophobic rat. It was Calvin Hall who first attempted to formally demonstrate the validity of OFD as an index of emotional arousal: He showed that it decreased over days as animals became more familiar with the test situation and that it was negatively correlated with the animal's willingness to eat in the same situation (Hall, 1934). Additional support for the validity of OFD was later supplied by Broadhurst, who showed that OFD increased in concert with experimentally imposed increases in illumination level and white noise intensity (Broadhurst, 1957).

The Progress of Selection. The open-field test used by Broadhurst was circular, brightly lit, and had uniform white walls. The frequency of defecation in it was used as an index of an animal's level of emotionality. High- and low-scoring animals in the parental and subsequent generations were selected on the basis of their mean open-field defecation score on four, daily, 2-minute trials and bred with siblings to create the inbred Maudsley Reactive (MR) and Maudsley Non-Reactive (MNR) strains. As can be seen in Figure 5.1, the effect of genetic selection was rapid: compared with a mean OFD score of approxi-

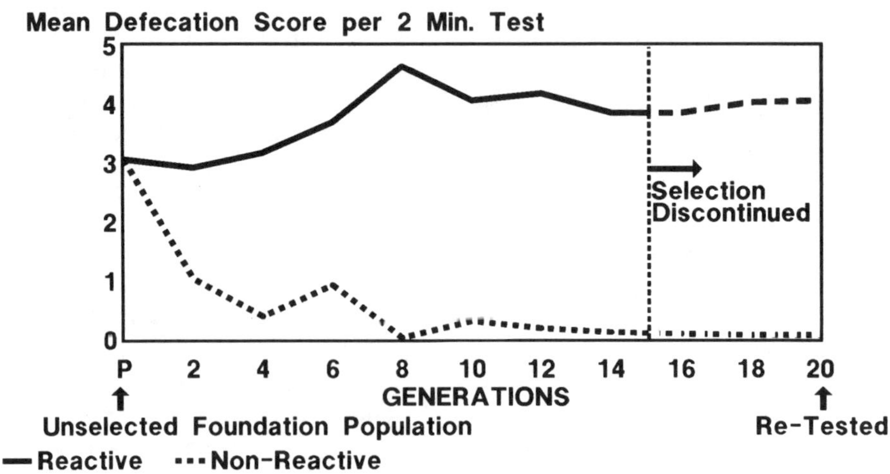

FIG. 5.1 Selection for open-field defecation in Maudsley Reactive and Non-Reactive rat strains (after Broadhurst, 1960, 1962).

mately three boli per trial in the parental population, MNR OFD scores approached zero by the fourth generation; by contrast, MR rats showed only a slight increase in OFD above that exhibited by the parental population. By generation 15 the differences in OFD in the Maudsley strains appeared to have reached asymptote. In addition, suspension of selection for five generations after generation 15 had no effect on the mean OFD score of MR and MNR strains when they were retested in generation 20. This observation is consistent with the hypothesis that the genetic system underlying variation in OFD in the strains is fixed within them. The selection study is described in detail by Broadhurst (Broadhurst, 1960, 1962) and has been reviewed in methodological perspective by the writer (Blizard, 1981).

The successful creation of the Maudsley strains confirmed the earlier work of Hall (Hall, 1938 1951). Hall genetically selected for variation in open-field defecation using a slightly different criterion, the number of days that rats defecated over 12 daily trials. As was the case in the Maudsley experiment, selection for decreased OFD was immediate, OFD scores approaching zero in the first generation, whereas selection for increased OFD was gradual not reaching asymptote until the ninth generation of selection. Taken together, the selection experiments clearly demonstrate that there is substantial genetic variation in open-field behavior and that it is subject to selection pressure. The demonstration of substantial variation in OFD across unselected inbred strains of rats (Harrington, 1972, 1979) and mice (Thompson, 1953) provides additional evidence of the contribution of genetic factors to variation in open-field behavior.

Genetic Variation in Other Psychophysiological Characteristics. Genetic contributions to individual differences in psychophysiological reactivity to stress have been found to be the rule rather than the exception. At the physiological level, strain differences have been demonstrated in cardiac reactivity to environmental stressors among inbred mice (Blizard & Welty, 1971) and twin studies have shown the existence of genetic influences on this trait in man (Carroll, Hewitt, Last, Turner, & Sims, 1985). Strain differences have been found in active avoidance behavior among mice (Collins, 1964) and rats (Harrington, 1981) and selection procedures have been successfully applied to this trait to create the Roman High- and Low-avoidance strains (Bignami, 1965). Social behaviors, like aggression, have also been demonstrated to be strain dependent (Scott, 1942), and selection procedures have been successfully applied to different aspects of aggressive behavior (Cairns, MacCombie, & Hood, 1983; Hyde & Sawyer, 1980; Lagerspetz, 1964).

Some evidence suggests that there is a correlation between psychophysiological response to social and nonsocial stimuli: Hall and Klein (1942) found male rats from Hall's line selected for low emotionality (low defecating) to be significantly more aggressive than those from the emotional line (high defecating). Reciprocally, mice of Lagerspetz's aggressive line defecated significantly less in the open-field than mice from her nonaggressive line (Lagerspetz, 1964). In both instances, increased aggressive tendencies were associated with decreased levels of open-field defecation. More research needs to be conducted in this area but it appears likely, on the basis of the earlier findings, that results obtained using the Maudsley strains which have been genetically selected for differences in open-field defecation may have relevance to the organism's response to a wide variety of social and environmental stimuli.

Transfer of the Maudsley Strains to the United States. The Maudsley strains were transferred to the United States in 1962 to Dr. Carl Hansen at NIH and in 1965 to Dr. Gordon Harrington at the University of Northern Iowa (Fig. 5.2). The different derivations of the Maudsleys have been assigned idiosyncratic genetic designations to distinguish them from each other and from the British stocks. The Maudsley strains maintained at the NIH are designated MR/N and MNR/N and those maintained by Harrington, the MR/Har, MNR/Har, and MNRA/Har strains. The two independent Non-Reactive strains that have been maintained at Northern Iowa differ at the agouti locus MNR/Har (AA) and MNRA/Har (aa) as well as in several other characteristics (see Blizard, 1981).

Both of the North American stocks of the Maudsleys have been found to differ reliably in open-field defecation provided they are tested under standardized conditions (Blizard, Hansen, & Freedman, 1982; Harrington & Blizard,

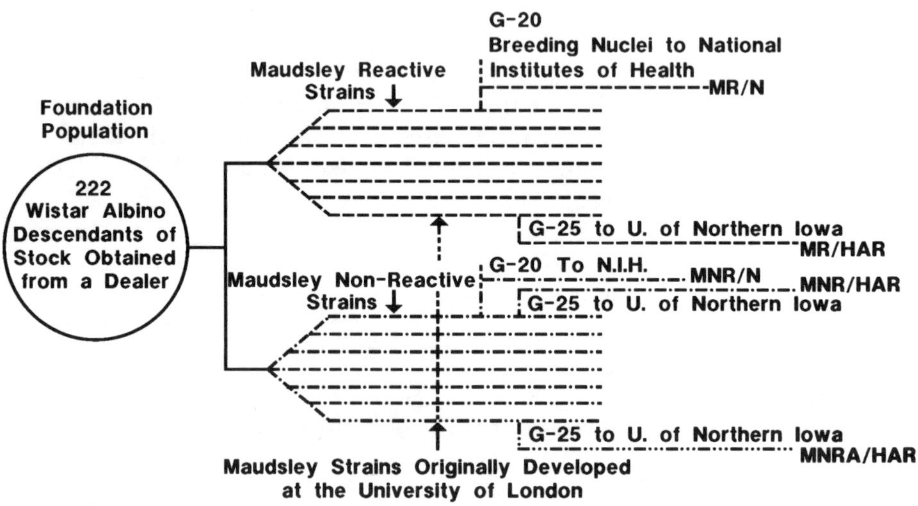

FIG. 5.2 Derivation of North American stocks of Maudsley Reactive and Non-Reactive strains.

1983). Thus, transfer of small breeding nuclei to the United States and maintenance without selection for some 40 generations of inbreeding has not disrupted the genetic system that is responsible for variations in OFD. The stability of expression of the differences in open-field defecation is an important advantage when using this particular genetic model. This, coupled to the high degree of inbreeding that has been achieved, ensures that a uniform and replicable genotype is available to researchers in different laboratories.

Correlates of Selection for OFD. During the process of selecting for variation in OFD, records were routinely kept of open-field activity (OFA). As selection proceeded, it became evident that the two strains were diverging on this characteristic with MR rats being less active in the open-field than MNRs (Fig. 5.3). The strain difference in OFA has also been found to be a consistent feature of the derivations of the Maudsleys that are maintained in North America (Blizard, 1981). In other words, genetic selection for variation in OFD has resulted in correlated selection for differences in OFA. Many other examples exist of responses that are correlated with OFD in the Maudsley model and have been summarized by Eysenck and Broadhurst (1964), and Broadhurst (1975). MR rats exhibit less efficient avoidance but faster escape than MNR rats in escape-avoidance conditioning (Levine & Broadhurst, 1963; Owen, 1963); greater suppression of bar pressing in a conditioned emotional response situation (Singh, 1959); and a greater increase in speed on frustrated trials in a double-runway frustration task (Savage & Eysenck, 1964). As noted, one of Broadhurst's prime goals in carrying out the selection experiment was to

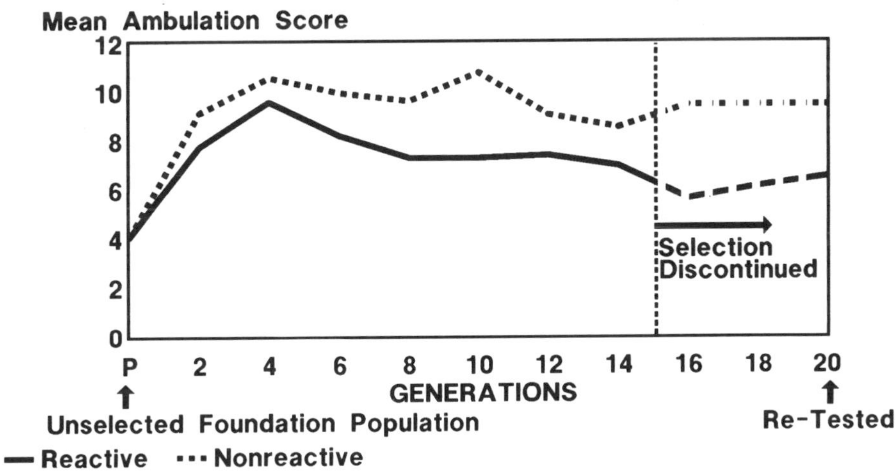

FIG. 5.3 Open-field activity in MR and MNR strains during selection for open-field defecation (after Broadhurst, 1960, 1962).

discover the impact of variations in emotionality upon particular patterns of behavior. The discovery of differences between the Maudsley strains in a variety of stressful situations shows that genetic selection for variation in response to a brief, open-field test has indeed had generalized effects on behavior. A logical extension of this work is to delineate the alterations in the nervous system that result in differences in open-field defecation and to elucidate their role in more complex behaviors such as escape-avoidance conditioning. Later in this chapter I discuss research that bears on this issue.

In judging the significance of correlations between characters among inbred strains, one must be careful to distinguish true from spurious genetic correlations (i.e., to separate those characteristics that reflect the genetic system that controls OFD from those that are the result of the fortuitous fixation of unrelated alleles during the inbreeding process). The usual method of distinguishing true from spurious correlations in selection studies is to breed replicate or control lines (Defries, 1967). This option was not deliberately exercised in the Maudsley experiment, but the MNRA/Har strain referred to earlier has been maintained and inbred as an independent strain since the second generation of selection (Blizard, 1981; Broadhurst, 1960) and therefore constitutes a useful replicate of selection for decreased emotionality. Blizard and Liang (1979a) used it to question the reliability of the association between OFD and the central serotonergic system previously reported to exist in the Maudsleys by Sudak and Maas (1964) and, conversely, Liang and Blizard (1978) confirmed the reliability of the relationship between OFD and the peripheral sympathetic system originally discovered in the MR/Har and MNR/Har strains by Slater, Blizard, and Pohorecky (1977) by extending comparisons of MR/Har to the MNRA/Har strain.

PATHWAYS BETWEEN GENES AND BEHAVIORAL CHARACTERS

Direct Mediation. The discovery of genetic variation in a character such as OFD does not elucidate the way in which genes influence its phenotypic expression. One possibility is that the genes influence structures involved in a character's expression by their regulatory control of relevant proteins or enzymes. For OFD, these might well be those elements of the nervous system that influence intestinal and colonic motility such as the peripheral autonomic nervous system or higher CNS structures that modulate autonomic reflexes. Genes could also influence membrane structure of the intestine and alter its intrinsic motility. In other words, genes may produce genetic variation in a psychophysiological character by direct effects on structures involved in its expression. This may occur either in adult life or during periods of development when the nervous system is being laid down and when neurotransmitter systems are maturing.

Indirect Mediation. A second possible mechanism is that genes may produce phenotypic variations in a character in an indirect manner. For example, genes could conceivably alter the maternal environment in which the fetus and offspring develop and this change in the developmental environment could then produce long-lasting changes in the organism. In this view, the primary effect of the genes is on the global maternal environment and their effect on the offspring is indirect or secondary. This mode of mediation seems especially plausible when considering behavioral alterations because the nervous system is exquisitely sensitive to environmental alterations during early life.

Early Onset of Strain Differences in Open-Field Behavior. Regardless of whether phenotypic differences between the Maudsleys are directly or indirectly mediated, recent observations from the writer's laboratory suggest that the differences in OFD between them can be observed in young animals. Animals were tested in the open field in the standard manner beginning at 23 and 29 days of age. MR animals defecated significantly more than MNRA/Har animals at all ages (Table 5.1). These results show that the genes that control the strain differences in OFD in the Maudsleys exert their effect early in the life of the organism. Individual differences in psychophysiological reactivity to social stimuli in primates also emerge early in ontogeny (see Kagan et al. and Levine & Wiener, this volume) and the findings in the Maudsley model are compatible with the existence of a similar developmental pattern across a wide variety of mammalian species. The early emergence of differences in OFD between the Maudsleys does not favor direct or indirect modes of mediation. Powerful methodologies exist, for the exploration of indirect mediation in inbred strains and these are discussed in the next section.

TABLE 5.1
Open-Field Behavior in Young Rats of the Maudsley Reactive and Non-Reactive Strains

	Maudsley Reactive (*N* = 35)	*Maudsley Non-Reactive* (*N* = 29)
Open-field Activity	127.9 ± 8.5	146.7 ± 7.82
Open-field Defecation	12.1 ± 1.1	0.4 ± 0.2

Note: Young rats (23–29 days old on the first day of testing) of the Maudsley Reactive (MR/Har) and Maudsley Non-Reactive (MNRA/Har) strains were tested for 2 minutes per day in a brightly illuminated open-field test for 4 consecutive days. The scores are total open-field activity or defecation over the four daily trials (Mean ± S.E.). As shown, MR/Har rats defecated significantly more over the 4 days than MNRA/Har animals; the strains did not differ significantly in activity.

THE MATERNAL ENVIRONMENT

In mammals, the maternal environment consists of the period of prenatal existence in utero when development of the fetus is dependent on an adequate supply of nutrients via its placental system and the period of postnatal life when the offspring are dependent on their mother for food, warmth, and protection. Experimental designs have been developed that permit independent examination of the effects of pre- and postnatal maternal influences when considering strain differences in behavior. These have been described by Broadhurst (1961) and are depicted in Table 5.2.

The Prenatal Environment. In the case of prenatal effects, the usual method is to carry out reciprocal crosses between two strains, nominally designated H and L in Table 5.2. Females of the L strain are mated with males of the H strain and, reciprocally, females of the H strain are mated with L males and their offspring are compared. The logic of this design is that the offspring of reciprocal crosses between inbred strains should be genetically identical because of the uniform heterozygosity of F1s. Any differences between them in the direction of the female parent may therefore be due to the differential effect of the intrauterine environments provided by the females of the two different strains. This, of course, assumes that postnatal effects are absent and that the results cannot be explained by sex linkage (discussed later).

The Postnatal Environment. Cross–fostering at birth is the method employed to evaluate the influence of the postnatal environment; offspring from an H mother are taken from her at birth and given to a mother from the L strain

TABLE 5.2
Experimental Design to Investigate the Contribution of Pre- and Postnatal Maternal Effects to Strain Differences in Behavior

Type of Effect	*Treatment*	*Mating-Scheme*			*Environment*	
		Female		Male	Prenatal	Postnatal
Prenatal	Reciprocal Crosses	H	X	L	H	H
		L	X	H	L	L
Postnatal	Cross-Fostering	H	X	H	H	L
		H	X	H	H	H
		L	X	L	L	H
		L	X	L	L	L

Note: H = a high-scoring strain, L = a low-scoring strain. The experimental designs for analysis of pre and postnatal effects are discussed in the text. Note that a completely rigorous design for the analysis of postnatal effects should include control groups to evaluate the effects of fostering (see text).

for rearing, and vice versa. Any postnatal effect can then be detected by comparing the scores of such fostered offspring with those that were not subjected to this change and who were reared by their natural mothers. If the offspring resemble the foster mother more than their natural mother, a postnatal maternal effect can be presumed. As a caveat, it is well known that fostering itself may have any effect on behavior and control groups may need to be included in the experimental design to examine for this possibility.

Sex Linkage and Maternal Mediation. When the reciprocal F1 methodology is used, sex linkage of a trait can produce a pattern of results that superficially resembles that produced by the prenatal environment. For example, when the F1 cross is carried out using an H mother and an L father, the resulting male offspring will receive an H–type X chromosome from the mother and an L–type Y chromosome from the father. The maternal environment in which F1 male offspring are raised (H) is thus confounded with the source of the X chromosome (H), the converse being true of the reciprocal cross. This confounding obviously does not apply to female offspring of reciprocal F1 crosses that carry an X chromosome of both H and L types. The reciprocal F1 methodology must therefore be used with care and the results carefully scrutinized to distinguish between sex linkage and a prenatal maternal influence. If a significant difference between reciprocal F1s is restricted to males then the possibility of sex linkage must be carefully evaluated. Research on this topic should therefore be of sufficient scope and design to evaluate the possibility involvement of sex linkage.

Cytoplasmic inheritance could also mimic prenatal effects in that the prenatal environment in reciprocal F1 crosses is confounded with the source of the ovum, the major contributor of cytoplasmic material. Although the possible contribution of cytoplasmic inheritance to phenotypic differences in behavior is hard to assess because of the paucity of available evidence, techniques such as transplantation of fertilized ova permit independent manipulation of prenatal environment and the source of the cytoplasm and should be considered in future studies.

MATERNAL CONTRIBUTIONS TO PHENOTYPIC DIFFERENCES AMONG THE MAUDSLEY STRAINS

Tests of the role of the pre- and postnatal environment on the differences in open-field behavior between the Maudsley strains were carried out by Broadhurst (1961). To examine for postnatal effects, complete litters were cross-fostered at birth between the two strains in the first six generations of selection and compared to unfostered controls. The offspring were all tested in the open-field in adult life in the standard manner. Cross-fostering had no effect on either OFD or OFA in either strain in any of the generations tested. The combined *N* over all generations for each strain was approximately 250, both in the fostered groups and also in those reared by their natural mother, the scope of the experiment lending confidence in its outcome. This experiment strongly suggests that differences in the open-field behavior of the two strains are independent of any differences that may exist in the postnatal maternal care of the mothers.

Prenatal influences on the strain differences in open-field behavior were examined by carrying out reciprocal crosses between Reactive and Non-Reactive strains in the sixth, seventh, and eighth generations of selection. It was found that F1 offspring born to Reactive mothers in the eighth generation of selection had significantly higher OFD scores than F1 offspring born to Non-Reactive mothers, but prenatal maternal environment had no significant effect on OFD in generations six and seven or when data were combined over all three generations. For OFA, the results provided stronger evidence of prenatal influences: In generation seven, F1 offspring born to Reactive mothers had significantly lower activity scores than offspring born to Non-Reactive mothers and a similar result was obtained when the data for generations six through eight were combined. As discussed earlier, MR rats have been consistently found to have a lower OFA than MNR animals and the fact that F1 offspring born to Reactive mothers have lower OFA than F1s born to Non-Reactive mothers is suggestive that prenatal influences contribute to one of the major indices of open-field behavior. Joffe (1965) later independently confirmed Broadhurst's principal findings.

More recently, I examined the effect of the prenatal maternal environment on open-field behavior in North American stocks of the Maudsley strains. MR/Har females were mated with MNR/Har males and vice versa to produce reciprocal F1 offspring. These offspring were then studied in the open-field in the standard manner. The results are shown in Table 5.3. As can be seen, F1 offspring, carried in utero in an MR/Har maternal environment, exhibited lower OFA than F1 offspring raised in an MNR/Har maternal environment. There were no differences in OFD between the reciprocal groupings. This small study on the Harrington stocks of the Maudsley strains is consistent with the results obtained separately by Broadhurst and Joffe. Thus, independent studies separated by more than 40 generations of inbreeding support the possibility that the prenatal maternal environment makes a contribution to differences in open-field activity in the Maudsley strains. Confirmation of the earlier findings suggests that they were not simply the result of transient alterations of the genome during the early part of the selection study, but were the result of genetic differences that are now fixed within the strains. The precise magnitude of the contribution made by the prenatal maternal environment to the phenotypic

TABLE 5.3
The Effect of Prenatal Maternal Environment on Open-Field Activity in Reciprocal F1 Crosses Between Maudsley Reactive (MR/Har) and Non-Reactive (MNR/Har) Strains

	Prenatal Maternal Environment	
	MR/Har	MNR/Har
F1 Male Offspring	157.4 ± 8.8	211.0 ± 11.1
	(N = 7)	(N = 12)
F1 Female Offspring	184.5 ± 8.3	212.0 ± 19.7
	(N = 6)	(N = 4)

Note: Total open-field activity over four daily, 2 minute tests (Mean ± S.E.) was compared in reciprocal F1 crosses between the Maudsley strains. F1 offspring raised by MR/Har mothers had significantly lower open-field activity when tested as adults than those raised by MNR/Har mothers ($p = < .005$, combining data from males and females). Because previous research has found no evidence of a postnatal maternal effect on OFA this result is consistent with the hypothesis that the different prenatal environments provided by MR/Har and MNR/Har mothers contribute to the well-established strain differences in open-field activity. There were no differences in open-field defecation between reciprocal F1 groupings. (See text for discussion of the experimental design.)

differences in open-field behavior is hard to determine; the earlier studies were done before the strain differences obtained by selection were stabilized, and the more recent investigations are too small in scale for satisfactory assessments to be made. The evidence suggests that the prenatal environment makes a major contribution to the strain differences in OFA but not to OFD. This is an important distinction because it would suggest that OFA and OFD are controlled by independent genetic systems.

MECHANISMS UNDERLYING PRENATAL INFLUENCES ON BEHAVIOR

A schema illustrating potential sources of mediation of prenatal influences on behavior is illustrated in Fig. 5.4. These may be from several different sources. (a) Originating in genetic differences between mothers: In this mode, the developing fetus may be exposed to a variety of genotype-dependent maternal hormonal influences. The Maudsley strains, for example, differ in thyroid (Feuer & Broadhurst, 1962) and adrenal (Feuer, 1963) status in adult life, and in a variety of other hormonal systems. Exposure of developing fetuses to different levels of trophic hormones could alter the rate of nervous system development and produce long-lasting changes capable of affecting adult behavior. In addition, systematic differences in the behavior of mothers, for example, in activity, could conceivably influence the course of development. (b) Environmental: consisting of random events experienced during the maternal period as well as systematic environmental differences such as exposure to a particular diet or toxic sub-

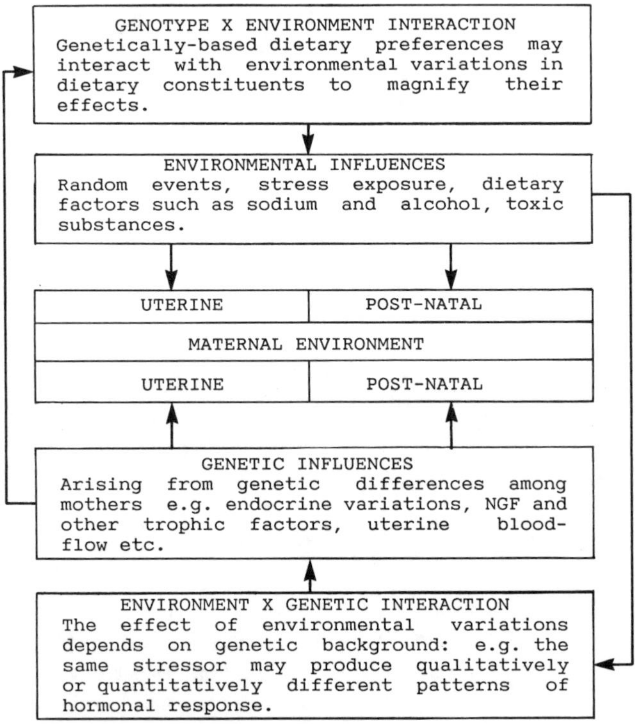

FIG. 5.4 Genetic and environmental influences during prenatal (uterine) and postnatal periods (until weaning) in mammals. (See text for discussion.)

stance. (c) Gene by environmental interactions: Genetic background may bias a mother toward a particular environmental stimulus and magnify its potential impact on offspring. Mothers of alcohol-preferring strains would belong in this category, in that, in an environment offering an opportunity to ingest ethanol, their offspring would be exposed to higher levels of ethanol than the offspring of mothers who do not prefer ethanol. (d) Environmental by genetic interaction: Reciprocally, an identical environmental stimulus could have a different impact on mothers of different genetic backgrounds. Exposure to trauma or stress, for example, could result in a qualitatively or quantitatively different pattern of endocrine arousal in different mothers and have potential impact on the maternal environment.

Prenatal influences on phenotypic differences between the Maudsley strains are likely to involve several of the pathways specified in Fig. 5.4. The only exception is that systematic environmental influences (described earlier in b) are unlikely to occur in a carefully controlled laboratory environment. In relation to genetic differences between mothers (see a), the many behavioral and biological differences that have been found between the Maudsley strains provide a valuable set of clues whose role in producing prenatal effects on behavior could be investigated.

In man, it is widely accepted that fetal development can be compromised by inadvertent exposure to drugs or toxic substances during pregnancy, but it is by no means established that variations in behavior in the normal range are influenced by subtle differences in the prenatal maternal environment. Nevertheless, the demonstration that systematic differences between the prenatal environment of Reactive and Non-Reactive mothers contribute to differences in OFA between the Maudsley strains suggests that similar influences should be carefully considered in research on man and other primates.

THE CNS AS A TARGET FOR GENE-ACTION IN THE MAUDSLEY STRAINS

Studies of the maternal environment are helpful in elucidating *the time* during which genetic influences on behavior have their impact but they do not delineate the somatic systems that are the target for gene-action. This is a difficult area of investigation because the organism's response to environmental and social stress is complex. It involves many levels of inquiry, including biochemical, endocrinological, physiological and behavioral responses, which interact with each other in subtle ways. These include activation of the hypothalamic–pituitary–adrenal axis, increased muscle tension due to supraspinal facilitation of alpha motoneurons, release of adrenaline from the adrenal medulla with its stimulatory effect on metabolism, and a variety of physiological changes mediated by the peripheral autonomic nervous system such as alterations in blood flow. These various changes are not isolated from each other but are carefully orchestrated to provide the organism with the resources to cope with a threatening situation in a coordinated manner. The circulatory changes involve redirection of blood flow to skeletal muscle that, as noted earlier, is in a heightened state of readiness for action. The simultaneous release of adrenaline that stimulates glycogenolysis also supports increased energy utilization.

The central nervous system undoubtedly plays an important role in the coordination or integration of the manifold physiological changes that accompany stress and thus it appears likely that selection for differences in OFD may be mediated by genetic influences on CNS-coordinating mechanisms. Although there are many loci which influence the organism's response to stress the central noradrenergic system is a prime candidate for consideration as a mediator of genetic influences on the brain. It is markedly activated by exposure to stress (Stone, 1975) and is believed to play an important role in the modulation of endocrine, behavioral, and physiological response. Among the various components of the central noradregenic system, the locus ceruleus (LC) is a likely focus of gene action. It projects to many areas of the central nervous system and its importance in these areas is demonstrated by the fact that lesions of it result in profound depletion of noradrenalin (NA) stores in cortex and other structures.

The Locus Ceruleus as a Stress Attenuator. The LC is exquisitely sensitive to chronic stress and it has been proposed that it exerts a stress-attenuating influence on the sequelae of chronic stress (Amaral & Sinnamon, 1977). Their view is based on observations of the relationship between the LC and a variety of physiological systems; its neurophysiological effects are consistent with its enhancing signal-to-noise ratio in the nervous systems; (Freedman, Hoffer, Woodward, & Puro, 1977); Its inhibitory effects via descending projections on the peripheral sympathetic nervous system (PSNS) (Snyder & Reis, 1975); and its restraining influence on hormones released during stress (reviewed by Amaral & Sinnamon, 1977). These effects of the LC have been proposed to enhance the organism's ability to deal with prepotent stimuli in the environment and enhance the organism's coping ability.

Evidence That the LC Mediates Phenotypic Differences Among the Maudsleys. To test the hypothesis that genetic differences between the Maudsley strains are mediated by variations in the LC, comparisons of LC-response to chronic stress were made by measuring tyrosine hydroxylase (TH) activity in the LC of the Maudsley strains under control and chronically stressed conditions (Blizard, Freedman, & Liang, 1983). This index was selected because TH is rate limiting in the biosynthesis of NA and thus alterations in its activity are likely to have significant neurochemical and neurophysiological effects. Invoking the hypothesis that the LC plays a stress-attenuating role (Amaral & Sinnamon, 1977), it was predicted that MNRA/Har rats, selectively bred for decreased stress-susceptibility, would exhibit a greater elevation in cerulear TH activity after chronic stress than MR/Har rats, selectively bred for heightened reactivity to stress. Accordingly, groups of Reactive and Non-Reactive male rats were exposed to a daily stress consisting of 50 minutes of exposure to intermittent foot-shock and were sacrificed approximately 24 hours after the ninth daily stress exposure. As shown in Fig. 5.5, exposure to this stressful regime, produced a significantly greater elevation of cerulear TH-activity in MNRA/Har than MR/Har male rats. Although not shown in Fig. 5.5, the greater elevation of cerulear TH in MNRA/Har rats was seen in three independent experiments, thus establishing it as a highly reliable strain difference. By comparison, the response of hypothalamic TH to chronic stress was small in magnitude and did not differ between the strains indicating that strain differences in the central noradrenergic system were regionally specific.

It is well established that repetitive application of a variety of stressors

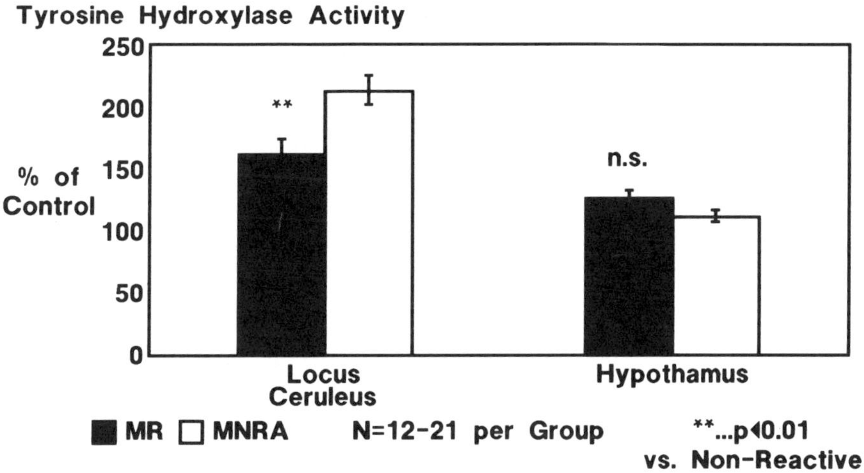

FIG. 5.5 Effects of chronic stress on tyrosine hydroxylase activity in two brain regions in the Maudsley Reactive (MR) and Maudsley Non-Reactive (MNRA) strains (after Blizard, Freedman, & Liang, 1983).

produces a delayed but long-lasting elevation in the activity of TH in the central and perhipheral noradrenergic systems (Zigmond, Schon, & Iversen, 1974). The stimulus for the increase in enzyme activity is believed to be the depletion of neuronal NA that follows acute stress (Weiss, Glazer, & Pohorecky, 1976), a possibility supported by the observation that the depletion and temporal recovery of tissue NA that follows reserpine administration is inversely correlated with the magnitude of TH-elevation (Reis, Joh, & Ross, 1975). Our explanation of the differential increase in TH activity in the two strains after chronic stress is that exposure to foot shock produced greater neuronal activity in the cerulear pathway of Non-Reactive rats, a correspondingly greater depletion of neuronal NA levels in this strain and hence, as outlined earlier, a stronger stimulus for enzyme induction in the LC of Non-Reactive rats.

The greater elevation of cerulear TH activity seen in Non-Reactive rats after chronic stress could afford enhanced protection against stress-induced NA depletion in several ways: by protecting animals against stress-induced NA depletion, by repleting NA stores more swiftly after stress, or by increasing NA stores above control levels thus providing greater reserve capacity in the noradrenergic system. All of these characteristics could conceivably enhance the ability of the central noradrenergic system to respond appropriately when it is subjected to increased demand, for example, in acute stress situations. Chronic stress also produced strain-dependent alterations in the peripheral noradrenergic system. After chronic stress, MNRA/Har rats exhibited increases and MR/Har rats no change in NA concentrations of small intestine and submaxillary gland. These differences demonstrate that strain-dependent variations in cerulear response to chronic stress are correlated with alterations in the PSNS which may have significance for autonomic response to stress.

It was argued earlier that the LC may bias the central nervous system to cope with phasically imperative events by enhancing signal-to-noise ratio in the nervous system (Amaral & Sinnamon, 1977). If exposure to foot shock does result in greater arousal of the cerulear pathway in Non-Reactive compared with Reactive rats, this could provide an attractive neuroanatomical basis for understanding the differential performance of the Maudsley strains in escape-avoidance conditioning (Levine & Broadhurst, 1963). For example, Non-Reactive rats avoid signalled electric shocks more efficiently than Reactive rats and this is consistent with their greater cerulear activation producing an enhanced signal-to-noise ratio in the nervous system thus facilitating attention and response to the warning stimulus. Greater cerulear activation in Non-Reactive rats may also be responsible for strain differences in conditioned emotional response (Singh, 1959), and other stressful behavioral tasks (Savage & Eysenck, 1964).

Amaral and Sinnamon's characterization of the LC as a stress-attenuating CNS-locus is based on evidence that suggests it plays a role in regulating autonomic as well as neurophysiological and behavioral response to stress. There is also much evidence that the Maudsley strains differ in autonomic function. Chronologically, this evidence was obtained before the studies on the LC were conducted, but it assumes special significance now that strain differences in cerulear function have been identified. Because this research has recently been reviewed elsewhere (Blizard, 1988), it is only briefly summarized here.

Diminished Reactivity of PSNS of Non-Reactive Rats to Acute Stress. As noted, Amaral and Sinnamon suggested that the LC exerts an inhibitory influence on the PSNS. Hence, it would be predicted that the Non-Reactive strain with its hypothesized greater cerulear reactivity to stress would exhibit diminished PSNS-reactivity to acute stress. Comparisons of plasma catecholamines under basal and stressful conditions support this proposition. Reactive rats exhibited significant increases in plasma NA and adrenalin (A) after three different stressors (handling, open-field exposure and immobilization) whereas Non-Reactive rats did not exhibit a significant increase in NA after any of the stressors and only showed a significant increase in A after open-field and immobilization tests (Blizard & Liang, 1979b). The strain difference did not simply reflect variation in the time-course of PSNS-response because the sampling times for the three tests ranged from 30 secs (Handling) to 5 min (Immobilization) following imposition of the stress. The fact that three different acute stresses produced a significant increase in NA in Reactive rats, but no significant change in Non-Reactive rats, suggests a generalized diminution in the reactivity of the PSNS in the Non-Reactive strain and is consistent with their greater cerulear reactivity described above.

Comparisons of cardiovascular reactivity to stress in the Maudsley strains also support the notion of diminished PSNS-reactivity in the Non-Reactive strain. Blizard (1968, 1971) compared HR-reactivity of Reactive and Non-Reactive rats to the auditory and visual stimuli used in the open-field test (white-noise and bright light). Non-Reactive rats showed smaller increments in HR than Reactive rats in response to these stimuli and also had slower HR after handling. A smaller increment in HR in response to a stressor is consistent with diminished release of NA and is therefore consistent with the Non-Reactive strain possessing attenuated PSNS-reactivity.

THE LOCUS CERULEUS AS A TARGET FOR GENE ACTION IN THE MAUDSLEY STRAINS

Amaral and Sinnamon argued that the LC exerts a stress-attenuating role in the nervous system whose influence would be seen at a variety of levels; in behavioral response to stressful situations, in effects on the peripheral sympathetic nervous system, and in endocrine response to stress. Utilizing this framework, it has been hypothesized that the LC has been a target for gene action in the Maudsley model. Three different lines of evidence support this hypothesis. First, the biochemical response of the LC to chronic stress differs in the Maudsley strains: I have suggested that the greater elevation of TH in the LC of Non-Reactive rats following chronic stress reflects a more profound activation of the cerulear pathway in Non-Reactive animals. Second, it has been argued that cerulear activation enhances the signal-to-noise ratio in the nervous system and biases the animal to respond to prepotent stimuli. Here, the marked behavioral differences in stressful situations in the Maudsley strains is consistent with this role of the LC. Third, the diminished PSNS-response of Non-Reactive rats to acute stress is also compatible with their possessing heightened cerulear activity because the LC is believed to exert a restraining influence on PSNS-activity.

The possibility that the LC is a focus of gene action in the Maudsley model has important heuristic value. It permits the various behavioral, biochemical, physiological, and endocrinological differences between the strains to be understood as being the result of a gene action at a particular locus in the nervous system. The LC has been the subject of intense investigation in recent years and the accumulation of knowledge about the LC endows great flexibility on future experimental approaches. Reciprocally, if future research continues to support involvement of the LC in the mediation of genetic differences between the

Maudsleys, this model may assist in the elucidation of the role this noradrenergic nucleus plays in mediating individual differences in the organism's response to uncertainty and stress.

Alterations in the Basal or Resting State of the PSNS in the Maudsley Strains. Although the differences in PSNS-reactivity between the Maudsley strains are most relevant to the alterations in cerulear function that have been discussed, differences in PSNS-state under basal conditions have also been discovered in this genetic model. These are briefly reviewed to provide complete information about the nature of alterations in PSNS-activity between the Maudsley strains.

Under basal or resting conditions, Non-Reactive rats have higher concentrations of catecholamines in a variety of peripheral tissues including heart, spleen, and adrenals (see Fig. 5.6; Liang & Blizard, 1978; Slater, Blizard, & Pohorecky, 1977) and submaxillary gland, small intestine, and colon (Blizard, Altman, & Freedman, 1982). These strain differences were found to be correlated with significant strain variations in plasma levels of NA under resting conditions with Non-Reactive rats having higher levels of NA than Reactive rats (Blizard, Liang, & Emmel, 1980). The higher basal level of NA in Non-Reactive rats is consistent with their possessing an elevated sympathetic tone (see Fig. 5.7). This interpretation is furthermore consistent with the discovery of a negative correlation between the plasma NA levels of the Maudsley strains and cardiac beta-receptor concentrations. Non-Reactive rats with the higher concentration of tissue and

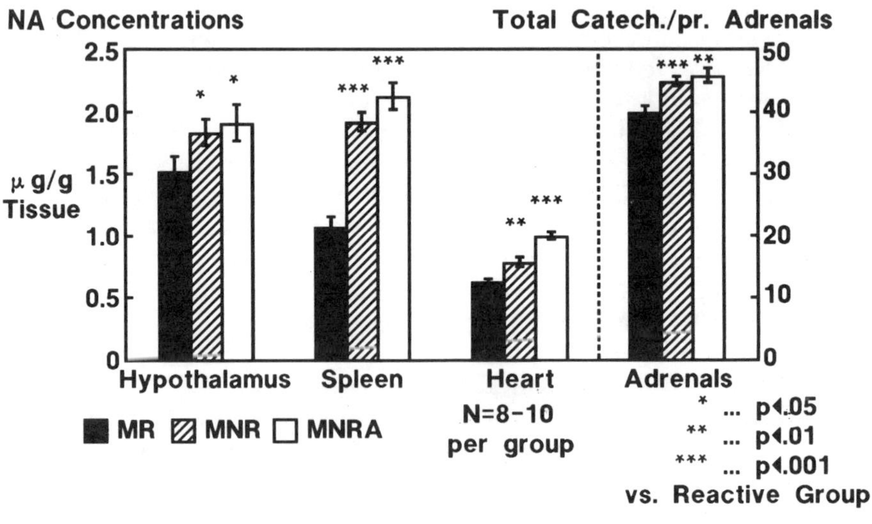

FIG. 5.6. Central and peripheral norepinephrine noradrenaline (NA) concentrations in the Maudsley strains (after Blizard & Liang, 1978).

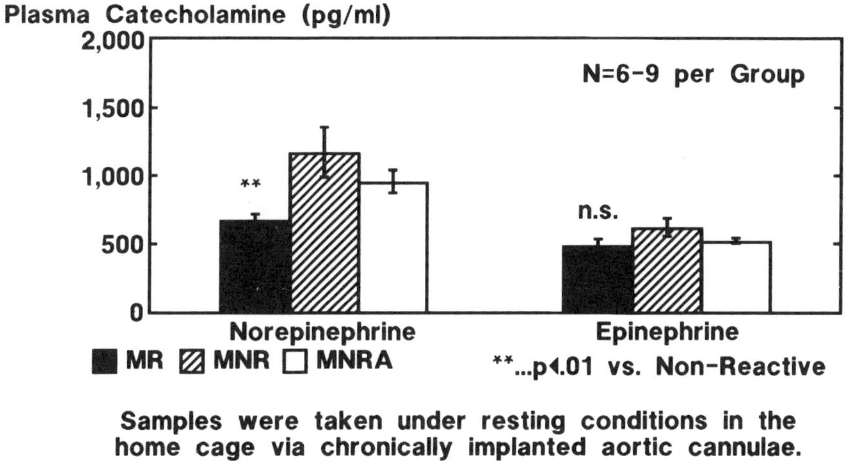

FIG. 5.7 Basal catecholamine levels inthe Maudsley strains (from Blizard, Liang, & Emmel, 1980).

plasma NA under resting conditions have lower concentrations of cardiac beta-receptors (Christ, Dunlap, & Blizard, 1988; Liang, Dunlap, Freedman, & Blizard, 1982). Up- and down-regulation of receptor populations in response to pharmacological manipulations is a well-established phenomenon (Mickey, Tate, Mullikin, & Lefkowitz, 1976; Sporn, Hardin, Wolfe, & Molinoff, 1976) and the negative correlation of agonist and cardiac beta-receptor in the Maudsley strains is consistent with the notion that exposure to the higher level of endogenous agonist in Non-Reactive animals produces a down-regulation of beta receptors.

These studies of the interrelationship of plasma catecholamines and cardiac beta receptors in the Maudsleys are of methodological significance for studies of the biological underpinnings of individual differences in behavior in man. It is clear that such inquiries should address the question of the status of relevant receptor populations as well as measurements of hormone or neurotransmitter levels. Unless information about the status of both the hormone *and* receptor concentrations are available it is difficult to speculate effectively about the direction and intensity of biological response.

Basal Alterations in Cardiovascular Function in the Maudsley Strains. The differences in the PSNS in the Maudselys under resting conditions extend to differences in cardiovascular function. Comparisons of HR and BP from chronically cannulated animals in their home cage revealed that MR/Har rats had higher systolic and diastolic BP and HR than Non-Reactive rats (see Fig. 5.8; Blizard, Liang, & Emmel, 1980). This finding appears para-

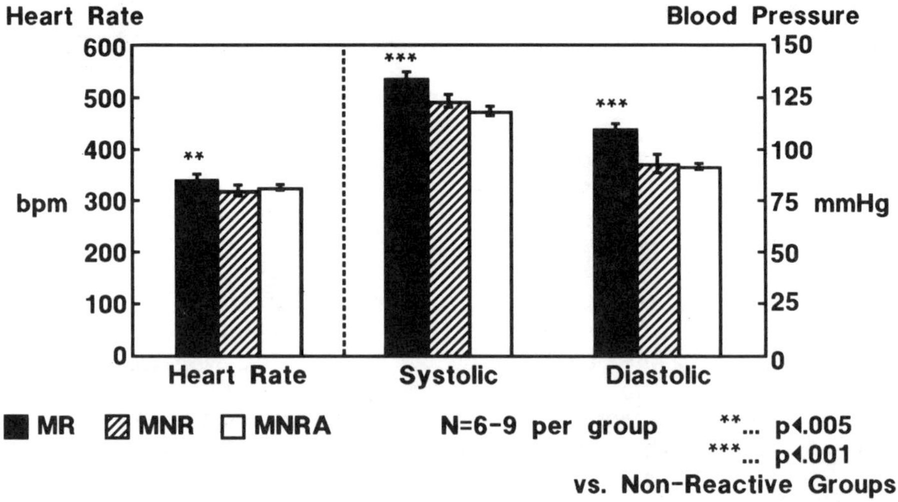

FIG. 5.8 Heart rate and blood pressure in the Maudsley strains under resting conditions (after Blizard, Liang, & Emmel, 1980).

doxical in that Reactive rats with their lower plasma levels of NA, an agonist that exerts a cardio-acceleratory and pressor influence, have higher BP and HR. The differences in receptor function described earlier may help resolve the paradox. The increased density of beta-receptors in MR/Har rats may compensate for the decreased levels of circulating NA and explain the higher resting HR and BP of MR/Har rats.

SIGNIFICANCE OF INDIVIDUAL DIFFERENCES IN BASAL AND REACTIVE STATES

Clearly, the differences between the Reactive and Non-Reactive strains encompass both reactive, and resting or basal dimensions. The Non-Reactive strain with the diminished PSNS-response to acute stress is characterized by greater sympathetic tone under resting conditions. The mechanisms underlying these strain differences may be interrelated. For example, according to Wilder's law of initial value (Wilder, 1962), a system's response potential is dependent upon the resting level of the system; for stimuli that increase a function, a high basal level reduces response magnitude, the converse applying to stimuli that decrease a function. Thus, the inability of acute stress to augment NA-release in Non-Reactive rats may be dependent on the high rate of release of NA under resting conditions. From a broader perspective, the distinction between basal and reactive states of the organism has obvious importance for human studies. In the analysis of the physiological and endocrine basis of individual variations in coping with social uncertainty in man and other primates it is especially important to distinguish between basal and reactive dimensions. Unless this is attempted the fundamental mechanisms underlying the relevant psychobiological constellations will not be elucidated.

OVERVIEW

Gene Action and the Nervous System. As discussed elsewhere in this volume, coping with social uncertainty engages a variety of biological systems. The research on the Maudsley model also illustrates the multi-layered complexity of the organism's response to stress. We have suggested that many of the variations in somatic response to stress can be understood as being the result of gene action at a defined locus in the nervous system. This approach enables one to understand the various components of the body's response to uncertainty as being the result of variations in a specific physiological pathway. This is a great advantage because it permits a relatively precise hypothetical approach to fundamental mechanisms and is therefore a valuable complement to studies which emphasize the correlational approach to understanding the constellation of biological changes associated with uncertainty. Although we have emphasized the potential role of the locus ceruleus in influencing the body's response to stress it is highly likely that gene action affects a large number of CNS-structures. The present focus on a single structure merely reflects the limited nature of our present knowledge.

Use of Inbred Strains to Circumvent Measurement Error. Many of the hormonal and physiological responses that are of interest to the student of individual differences are characterized by great lability. For example, the plasma concentration of a hormone may be measured at a fixed time after exposure to a specific stimulus. The concentration of the hormone is influenced by a variety of sources of variation many of which are connected with the difficulty of obtaining a sample in a stress-free manner, as well as any variation in the manner in which the individual is exposed to the test stimulus. Thus, an individual's hormone index consists of the unique aspects of that individual as well as substantial sources of measurement error that have been exemplified previously. This is a considerable problem when correlations between different indices are calculated: Obviously, a statistically significant group correlation can result from measurement errors in one or two subjects. Also, biologically meaningful correlations can be obscured in the same way.

The use of inbred strains can avoid this problem because it permits the replication of a specific genotype (or individual) as many times as the experimenter wishes so that the experimenter can accurately determine that genotype's score. The same sources of variation still contribute to each subject's score but these variations are assumed to vary equally in a positive and negative direction and therefore not bias the final determination of the true mean associated with the particular genotype of interest. This issue is discussed in more detail in Blizard and Bailey (1979).

Genetic Methods Permit Examination of the Prenatal Environment. Our review of research on the Maudsley strains has also shown that prenatal influences that are under genetic control contribute to phenotypic variation in open-field activity. This demonstration shows that prenatal influences can contribute to behavior within the normal range and opens up this period of development for empirical study. The special experimental designs that were described earlier that permit examination of pre- and postnatal influences illustrate the power of genetic manipulations to study the sources of individual variation. Only additional experimentation will reveal whether prenatal influences contribute to other phenotypic differences between the Maudsley strains or individual differences in behavior in man.

ACKNOWLEDGMENT

Preparation of this chapter was supported in part by NIMH grant by MH-39210 to the author.

REFERENCES

Adams, N. & Blizard, D. A. (1987). Defeat and cardiovascular response. *The Psychological Record, 37*, 349–368.

Amaral, D. G., & Sinnamon, H. M. (1977). The locus coeruleus: neurobiology of a central noradrenergic nucleus. *Progress in Neurobiology, 9*, 147–196.

Aston-Jones, G., & Bloom, F. E. (1981). Norepinephrine-containing locus coeruleus neurons in behaving rats exhibit pronounced responses to non-noxious environmental stimuli. *Journal of Neuroscience, 1*, 887–900.

Bignami, G. (1965). Selection for high rates and low rates of conditioning in the rat. *Animal Behaviour, 13*, 221–227.

Blizard, D. A. (1968). *Autonomic and behavioral correlates of emotionality.* Unpublished doctoral thesis, University of Wales, Cardiff.

Blizard, D. A. (1971). Autonomic reactivity in the rat: Effects of genetic selection for emotionality. *Journal of Comparative Physiological Psychology, 76*, 282–289.

Blizard, D. A. (1981). The Maudsley Reactive and Non-Reactive strains: a North American perspective. *Behavior Genetics, 11*, 469–489.

Blizard, D. A. (1988). The locus ceruleus: A possible neural focus for genetic differences in emotionality, *Experientia, 44*, 491–495.

Blizard, D. A., Altman, H. J., & Freedman, L. S. (1982). The peripheral sympathetic nervous system in rat strains selectively bred for differences in response to stress. *Behavioral and Neural Biology, 34*, 319–325.

Blizard, D. A., & Bailey, D. W. (1979). Genetic correlation between open-field activity and defecation analysis with CXB recombinant-inbred strains. *Behavior Genetics, 9*, 349–357.

Blizard, D. A., Freedman, L. S., & Liang, B. (1983). Genetic variation, chronic stress, and the central and peripheral noradrenergic systems. *American Journal of Physiology, 245*, R600–R605.

Blizard, D. A., & Fulker, D. W. (1981). Rattus norvegicus as a tool in mammalian behavior genetics. *Behavior Genetics* (Whole Volume *11*,5).

Blizard, D. A., Hansen, C. T., & Freedman, L. S. (1982). Open-field behavior and theperipheral sympathetic nervous system in the MR/N and MNR/N rat strains. *Behavior Genetics, 12*, 459–466.

Blizard, D. A., & Liang, B. (1979a). Central serotonergic function and behavior in the Maudsley Reactive and Nonreactive strains: a reevaluation. *Behavior Genetics, 9*, 413–418.

Blizard, D., A., & Liang, B. (1979b). Plasma catecholamines under basal and stressful conditions in rat strains selectively bred for differences in response to stress. In E. Usdin (Ed.), *Catecholamines: Basic and clinical frontiers* (Proceedings of the 4th International Catecholamine Symposium). New York: Pergamon Press.

Blizard, D. A., Liang, B., & Emmel, D. K. (1980). Blood pressure, heart rate and plasma catecholamines under resting conditions in rat strains selectively bred for differences in response to stress. *Behavioral and Neural Biology, 29*,487–492.

Blizard, D. A., & Welty, R. (1971). Cardiac activity in the mouse: strain differences. *Journal of Comparative and Physiological Psychology, 77*, 337–344.

Broadhurst, P. L. (1956). *Emotionality in the rat a study of its determinants, inheritance and relationship to some aspects of motivation.* Unpublished doctoral thesis, University of London.

Broadhurst, P. L. (1957). Determinants of emotionality in the rat: I. Situational factors. *British Journal of Psychology, 48*, 1–12.

Broadhurst, P. L. (1960). Experiments in psychogenetics: Applications of biometrical genetics to the inheritance of behavior. In H. J. Eysenck (Ed.), *Experiments in personality: Vol. 1, Psychogenetics and psychopharmacology, (pp. 1–102).* London: Routledge and Kegan Paul.

Broadhurst, P. L. (1961). Analysis of maternal effects in the inheritance of behavior, *Animal Behaviour, 9*, 3–4.

Broadhurst, P. L. (1962). A note on further progress in a psychogenetic selection experiment. *Psychological Reports, 10*, 65–66.

Broadhurst, P. L. (1975). The Maudsley Reactive and Non-Reactive strains of rats. *Behavior Genetics, 5*, 299–319.

Cairns, R. B., MacCombie, D. J., & Hood, K. E. (1983). A developmental–genetic analysis of aggressive behavior in mice: I. Behavioral outcomes. *Journal of Comparative Psychology, 97*, 69–89.

Carroll, D., Hewitt, J. K., Last, K. A., Turner, J. R., & Sims, J. (1985). A twin study of cardiac reactivity and its relationship to parental blood pressure, *Physiology and Behavior, 14*, 103–106.

Christ, G. J., Dunlap, C. E., & Blizard, D. A. (1988). Genetic influences on agonist-binding to cardiac beta-receptors. *Biochemical Pharmacology, 37*, 1281–1286.

Collins, R. L. (1964). Inheritance of avoidance conditioning in mice: a diallel study, *Science, 103*, 1188–1190.

Defries, J. C. (1967). Quantitative genetics and behavior: overview and perspective. In J. Hirsch (Ed.), *Behavior-genetic analysis* (pp. 322–339). New York: McGraw-Hill.
Eysenck, H. J. (1967). *The biological basis of personality*. Springfield, IL: Charles C. Thomas
Eysenck, H. J., & Broadhurst, P. L. (1964). Experiments with animals: Introduction. In H. J. Eysenck (Ed.), *Experiments in motivation* (pp. 285–291). Oxford: Pergamon.
Feuer, G. (1963). Adrenal cortical activity and stress–response in rats selectively bred for differences in behavior. *Journal of Physiology, 169*, 43–44.
Feuer, G., & Broadhurst, P. L. (1962). Thyroid function in rats selectively bred for differences in emotional elimination. I. Differences in thyroid hormones. *Journal of Endocrinology, 24*, 127–136.
Freedman, R., Hoffer, B. J., Woodward, D. J., & Puro, D. (1977). Interaction of norepinephrine with cerebellar activity evoked by mossy and climbing fibers. *Experimental Neurology, 55*, 269–288.
Hall, C. S. (1934). Emotional behavior in the rat. I. Defecation and urination as measures of individual differences in emotionality. *Journal of Comparative Psychology, 18*, 385–403.
Hall, C. S. (1938). The inheritance of emotionality. *Sigma Xi Quarterly, 26*, 17–27.
Hall, C. S. (1951). The genetics of behavior. In S. S. Stevens (Ed.), Handbook of experimental psychology (pp. 304–329). New York: Wiley.
Hall, C. S., & Klein, S. J. (1942). Individual differences in aggressiveness in rats. *Journal of Comparative Psychology, 33*, 371–383.
Harrington, G. M. (1972). Strain differences in open-field behavior of the rat, *Psychonomic Science, 27*, 51–53.
Harrington, G. M. (1979). Strain differences in open-field behavior of the rat, II, *Bulletin of the Psychonomic Society, 13*, 85–86.
Harrington, G. M. (1981). The Har strains of rats: Origins and characteristics. *Behavior Genetics, 11*, 445–468.
Harrington, G. M., & Blizard, D. A. (1983). Open-field behavior in the Maudsley reactive and Non-Reactive strains: Procedural variations. *Behavior Genetics, 13*, 91–94.
Hyde, J. S., & Sawyer, T. F. (1980). Selection for agonistic behavior in wild female mice. *Behavior Genetics, 10*, 349–360.
Joffe, J. M. (1965). Genotype and prenatal and premating stress interact to affect adult behavior in rats. *Science, 150*, 1844–1845.
Lagerspetz, K. M. J. (1964). Studies on the aggressive behaviour of mice, *Annales Academiae Scientarum Fennicae, Series B., 131*,3, 1–131.
Levine, S., & Broadhurst, P. L. (1963). Genetic and ontogenetic influences on later emotionality in the rat. *Journal of Comparative and Physiological Psychology, 56*, 423–428.
Liang, B., & Blizard, D. A. (1978). Central and peripheral norepinephrine concentrations in rat strains selectively bred for differences in response to stress: confirmation and extension. *Pharmacology, Biochemistry and Behavior, 8*, 75–80.
Liang, B., Dunlap, C. E., Freedman, L. S., & Blizard, D. A. (1982). Variation in number and affinity of cardiac beta-receptors in the Maudsley reactive and non-reactive strains, *Life Sciences, 31*, 533–539.
Mickey, J. V., Tate, R. M., Mullikin, D., & Lefkowitz, R. J. (1976). Regulation of adenylate–cyclase coupled beta–adrenergic receptor binding sites by beta–ad-

renergic catecholamines in vitro. *Molecular Pharmacology, 12*, 409–419.

Owen, S. (1963). The effect on avoidance response extinction in rats of CS continuation and emotional constitution. *Journal of Genetic Psychology, 103*, 147–151.

Reis, D. J., Joh, T. H., & Ross, R. A. (1975). Effects of reserpine on activities and amounts of tyrosine hydroxylase and dopamine-hydroxylase in catecholamine neuronal systems in rat brain. *Journal of Pharmacology and Experimental Therapeutics, 193*, 775–783.

Savage, R. D., & Eysenck, H. J. (1964). The definition and measurement of emotionality. In H. J. Eysenck (Ed.), *Experiments in motivation* (pp. 292–314). Oxford: Pergamon Press.

Scott, J. P. (1942). Genetic difference in the social behavior of inbred strains of mice, *Journal of Heredity, 33*, 11–15.

Singh, S. D. (1959). Conditioned emotional response in the rat. I. Constitutional determinants. *Journal of Comparative and Physiological Psychology, 52*, 574–578.

Slater, J., Blizard, D. A., & Pohorecky, L. A. (1977). Central and peripheral norepinephrine metabolism in rat strains selectively bred for differences in response to stress. *Pharmacology, Biochemistry and Behavior, 6*, 511–520.

Snyder, D. W., & Reis, D. J. (1975). Sudden death following bilateral lesions of nucleus locus ceruleus, *Neuroscience Abstract, 1*, 425.

Sporn, J. R., Hardin, T. K., Wolfe, B. B., & Molinoff, P. B. (1976). Beta-adrenergic involvement in 6-hydroxydopamine induced supersensitivity in rat cerebral cortex. *Science, 194*, 624–626.

Stone, E. A. (1975). Stress and catecholamines. In A. J. Friedhoff (Ed.), *Catecholamines and Behavior* (Vol. 2) *Neuropsychopharmacology* (pp. 31–72). New York: Plenum Press.

Sudak, H. S., & Maas, J. W. (1964). Behavioral-neurochemical correlation in reactive and non-reactive rats. *Science, 46*, 418–420.

Thompson, W. R. (1953). The inheritance of behaviour: behavioral differences in fifteen mouse strains. *Canadian Journal of Psychology, 7*, 145–155.

Weiss, J. M., Glazer, H. I., & Pohorecky, L. A. (1976). Coping behavior and neurochemical changes: An alternative explanation for the original "learned helplessness" experiments. In A. Kling & G. Serban (Eds.), *Animal models in human psychobiology*, (pp. 141–173). New York: Plenum Press.

Wilder, J. (1962). Basimetric approach (law of initial value) to biological rhythms. *Annals of the New York Academy of Sciences, 98*, 1211–1221.

Zigmond, R. E., Schon, F., & Iversen, L. L. (1974). Increased tyrosine hydroxylase activity in the locus coeruleus of the rat brain after reserpine treatment and cold stress. *Brain Research, 70*, 547–552.

6

Coping With Uncertainty:
New Models of the Relations Between Hormonal, Behavioral, and Cognitive Processes

Megan Gunnar
Denny Marvinney
Jill Isensee
The Institute of Child Development
University of Minnesota

Robert O. Fisch
Department of Pediatrics
University of Minnesota

Philosophers of science have long been concerned with what constitutes an adequate disconfirmation of a theory or hypothesis (Kuhn, 1970). The history of science provides no easy answers. In some instances those who have championed an hypothesis in the face of disconfirming evidence have later been vindicated; in other instances they have not (Feyerabend, 1970; Popper, 1972). I am concerned here with the hypothesis that emotional distress or emotional arousal triggers the activation of the adrenocortical system. This hypothesis has been the basis of an enormous amount of research in the past several decades (see reviews by Gunnar, 1986a; Hennessy & Levine, 1979; Mason, 1959, 1968; Rose, 1980; Tennes & Mason, 1982). It developed out of studies that suggested that psychological factors serve as the final common pathway in what Selye had initially believed was a neuroendocrine nonspecific response to noxious stimulation (Mason, 1959). In this work, novelty, unpredictability, and strangeness were found to be common elements in stressful situations and it was argued that these variables activated the adrenocortical system via their effects on emotional state. Reviewing decades of research, Tennes and Mason (1982) concluded that "emotions have been established as a primary determinant of endocrine activity in human adults" (p. 21). Other reviewers, have echoed this conclusion (Frankenhaeuser, 1980; Gunnar, 1986a; Ursin, Baade, & Levine, 1978). Hennessy and Levine (1979) offered a somewhat different view, one that equated activation of the hypothalamic-pituitary-adrenocortical axis with arousal. However, whether arousal or emotional distress, the expectation clearly has been that measures of adrenocortical activity provide a window on the individual's inner state.

We have clung to this belief despite numerous instances of dissociations between behavioral measures of affect and arousal and plasma or urinary measures of cortisol. In fact, like believers who become more adamant when the predictions of the prophet fail, dissociations often increase, rather than decrease, our faith in cortisol as a measure of emotional arousal. For example, in an often cited study of parents of leukemic children, dissociations were found between parental expressions of distress and urinary 17-OHCS levels (Wolff, Hofer, & Mason, 1964). Rather than questioning the value of glucocorticoid metabolites as measures of emotional distress, the researchers sought alternative explanations for the dissociations. They argued that parents who appeared calm but had elevated cortisol levels were using denial as a defense, whereas parents who appeared distressed but had low cortisol levels were using hysterical behavior as a coping strategy. Similarly, in a study that was conducted with Gonzales, Goodlin, and Levine (Gunnar, Gonzales, Goodlin, & Levine, 1981a), it was argued that rhesus infants adapted to separation from their mothers within 24 hours because their cortisol levels by that time had returned to base; this despite the fact that behaviorally they continued to be highly agitated.

As noted at the outset, the history of science provides no simple guide for what to do when data do not appear to fit theory. When and whether to abandon a theory or hypothesis in many instances must be a judgment call; a judgment that often seems to be made only when the researcher is confronted by too many dissociations or too fundamental a contradiction in his or her own data. In what follows we describe the data that has led us to search for an alternative model, the model that we think better suits the evidence, and the value of this model to a developmental analysis of how children cope with uncertainty.

HORMONE-BEHAVIOR DISSOCIATIONS IN THE HUMAN NEWBORN

The disconfirming data were obtained from human newborns, in most cases newborns selected to conform to very stringent health criteria: normal gestational age, uneventful vaginal or repeat scheduled C-section deliver, 5 minute Apgar scores greater than 7 and normal neonatal course. Both behavioral and plasma cortisol measures were obtained while these newborns were responding to a variety of normally occurring events in the hospital nursery. Behavioral state was scored every 30 seconds using the state descriptors in Table 6.1. In all of the studies the newborns were followed for several hours prior to testing and any disturbing stimulation was avoided to help ensure low baseline or pretest

TABLE 6.1
Definitions of Behavioral States

State	*Descriptor*	*Definition*
1	Quiet sleep	Eyes shut, no REMs, regular respiration, no (or minimal) diffuse motor activity
2	Active sleep	Eyes shut, occasional REMs, irregular respiration, occasional gross motor activity
3	Drowsy	Eyes open and close, eyes look "dull," unfocused or "heavy," variable activity, spurts of writhing, may fuss slightly
4	Alert	Eyes open, "bright," focus on source of stimulation, minimal motor movement
5	Active awake	Eyes open but not shiny bright as in alert, high motor activity level with thrusting of extremities, may fuss but does not cry for sustained periods
6	Crying	Sustained crying (more than 15 sec)

cortisol levels. Over repeated studies our baseline levels have averaged between 2 and roughly 5 μg/dl using these procedures (Gunnar, Connors, Isensee, & Wall, 1988; Gunnar, Malone, Vance, & Fisch, 1985; Malone, Gunnar, & Fisch, 1985). In some studies, a baseline plasma sample was obtained immediately prior to initiating the "test" stimulation, in which case the stimulation was considered to include the blood sampling. In other studies, separate groups of newborns were used to determine baseline cortisol levels. Finally, in most of the studies posttest plasma samples were taken either 20 or 30 minutes after initiating the "test" event. In the initial studies, plasma was obtained via scalp vein sampling; in the later studies heel-stick sampling was used. In none of the studies did groups differ in behavioral state or plasma cortisol in the period immediately preceeding the test procedure.

In the first studies, we did not find dissociations (Gunnar, Fisch, Korsvik, & Donhowe, 1981b; Gunnar, Malone, Vance, & Fisch, 1985). We were studying newborns being circumcised and, in that context, elevations in plasma cortisol were positively correlated with behavioral distress (see Table 6.2). These results were consistent with those obtained previously by Anders, Sachar, Kream, Roffwarg, and Hellman (1970) and by Tennes and Carter (1973), and supported the idea that during the newborn period the adrenocortical response is "aroused by negative emotion manifested as crying" (Tennes & Mason, 1982, p. 26). We also found similar positive correlations between plasma cortisol and behavioral state using heel–stick blood sampling as the aversive stimulus (Gunnar, 1986b; Gunnar, Connors, Isensee, & Wall, 1988; see Table 6.2).

The first evidence of dissociation came in a study in which we attempted to modify the adrenocortical response to circumcision by soothing the newborn (nonnutritive sucking, stroking, and so on) during the surgery. As shown in Fig. 6.1, soothing effectively reduced behavioral distress, but had no effect on

TABLE 6.2
Plasma Cortisol and % Crying in Response to Circumcision and Heel–Stick Blood Sampling

Study	n	Stimulus	Time[a] Point	r
Gunnar et al., 1981b	9	Circumcision	30 min	+.71
Gunnar, Malone et al., 1985	20	Circumcision (w/soothing)[b]	30 min	+.44
Gunnar, Malone et al., 1985	20	Circumcision (w/soothing)	90 min	+.50
Gunnar, Connors, Isensee, & Wall, 1988	13	Circumcision (no soothing)	20 min	+.35
Gunnar, Connors, Isensee, & Wall, 1988	18	Heel-stick (no soothing)	20 min	+.54
Gunnar, 1986b	13	Heel-stick (w/soothing)	20 min	+.50
Gunnar, 1986b	12	Heel-stick (no soothing)	20 min	+.55

[a]Time point indicates minutes between onset of stimulation and poststimulation blood sampling. Behavior was always obtained during stimulation.

[b]Soothing indicates that all subjects were given pacifiers.

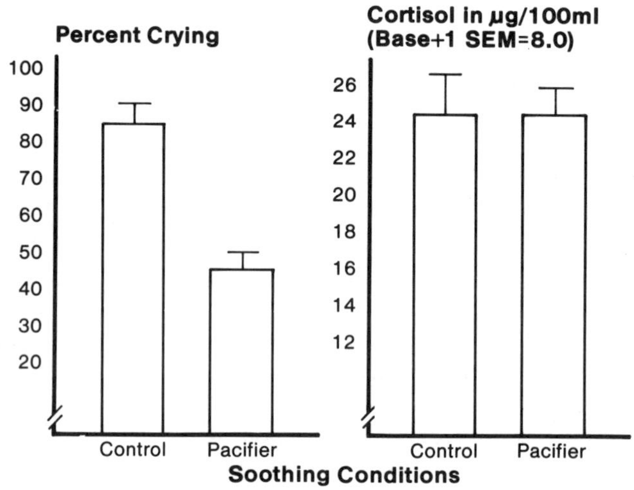

FIG. 6.1. The effects of soothing on behavioral and adrenocortical responses to routine circumcision without anesthesia in healthy human newborns (from Gunnar, Fisch, & Malone, 1984). Bars represent SEM.

postcircumcision plasma cortisol levels (Gunnar, Fisch, & Malone, 1984). As shown in Fig. 6.2, we found that soothing the newborn during a heel-stick blood draw in a subsequent study also reduced behavioral distress, but as before, failed to reduce the adrenocortical response (Gunnar, 1986a). We began to suspect that when the aversive stimulus involved pain or tissue damage the adrenocortical system was triggered through reflex neural pathways operating relatively independently of those pathways through which soothing interventions were modifying the behavioral response. This did not seem at the time a

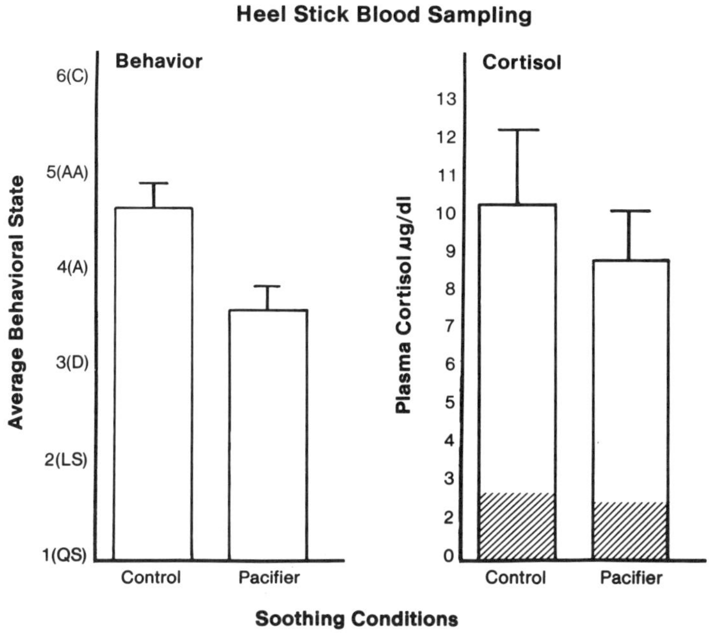

FIG. 6.2. The effects of soothing on responses to heel-stick blood sampling (from Gunnar, 1986b). Bar represent SEM. Hatched area reflect baseline cortisol levels.

serious challenge to the original hypothesis that emotional arousal, as reflected in behavioral state, was a primary trigger of the pituitary-adrenocortical system in the newborn.

However, in the same study in which we attempted to modify the adrenal response to blood sampling by soothing the babies, we attempted to do the same for newborns responding to a discharge examination (Gunnar, 1986b). Previously we had found that plasma cortisol levels following either weighing and measuring or a discharge exam were elevated to levels similar to those found following heel-stick blood sampling (Gunnar, Connors, Isensee, & Wall, 1988). Because we expected that the adrenal response to these normal caregiving interventions was largely mediated by the effects of these interventions on behavioral state, we expected that keeping the newborn calm would reduce, if not prevent, the adrenocortical response. However, as shown in Fig. 6.3, this was not the case. Soothing the newborn reduced behavioral arousal, but had no significant effect on the adrenocortical response to the discharge exam. Taken together, these results clearly indicated that, in the newborn, reducing behavioral arousal does not modify the adrenocortical response to either noxious or seemingly innocuous events. This posed a stronger challenge to the original hypothesis.

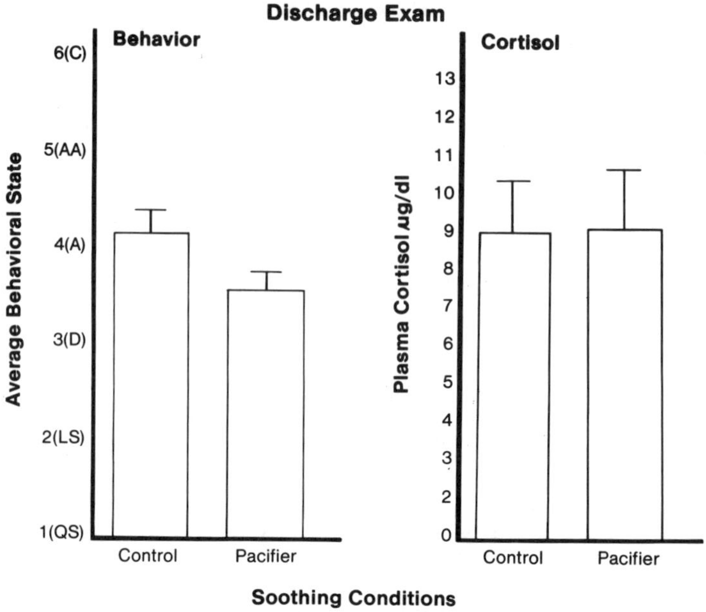

FIG. 6.3. The effects of soothing on responses to a discharge exam (from Gunnar, 1986b). Bars represent SEM.

Of even greater concern, however, were results obtained when we examined the correlations between behavioral state and plasma cortisol in response to normal caregiving manipulations. To our surprise, the pattern of relations was the opposite of what we had seen before. Distressed behavior was negatively correlated, and a derived measure of quiescent behavior was positively correlated with plasma cortisol (see Table 6.3). Thus, not only could we modify behavioral state without affecting the adrenal response to stimulation, but the direction of the correlation between behavioral state and plasma cortisol appeared to depend on the stimulus context. In response to noxious stimulation (circumcision and blood sampling) plasma cortisol elevations were positively correlated with greater behavioral arousal and distress; in response to seemingly innocuous caregiving interactions (weighing and measuring or a discharge examination) similar elevations in plasma cortisol were negatively correlated with behavioral arousal.

The newborns in all of the studies described here were extremely healthy. In one study, however, we did compare the behavioral and hormonal responses of extremely healthy newborns to those of newborns who exhibited "nonoptimal" signs (e.g., gestational age 36 to 37 weeks or over 42 weeks, fetal distress during delivery, low Apgars; Gunnar, Isensee, & Fust, in press) but were, nonetheless,

TABLE 6.3
Relations Between Crying vs. Quiescent Behavior and Plasma Cortisol in Response to Different Events in Healthy Newborns

			Correlation w/	
Stimulus	*n*	*Soothed*[a]	*% Crying*	*Quiescent Behavior*
Circumcision	6	no	+.35	−.53**
Blood sampling	18	no	+.54**	−.54**
Blood sampling	13	no	+.55**	−.04
Blood sampling	14	yes	+.50*	−.17
Weigh & measure	17	no	−.23	+.55**
Discharge exam	13	no	−.03	−.10
Discharge exam	12	no	−.52*	+.36
Discharge exam	12	yes	−.60**	+.61**

Note: Postsession plasma cortisol estimates obtained at 20 min (data are from Gunnar, Connors, Isensee, & Wall, 1988; Gunnar, 1986b).

[a]Soothed reflects use of pacifier

*$p < .10$

**$p < .05$

healthy enough to be cared for in a normal newborn nursery (see Table 6.4). We examined both groups with the Brazelton Neonatal Behavioral Assessment Scale, a commonly used assessment procedure that yields measures of behavioral arousal and behavioral organization (Brazelton, 1973). We expected that measures shown by others to load on a behavioral arousal or distress factor would be positively correlated with postBrazelton plasma cortisol levels for both groups of newborns. This was not the case. Although the two groups did not differ on either the behavioral or adrenocortical measures of response to the exam, and although both groups exhibited considerable variation in postBrazelton plasma cortisol levels, only in the "nonoptimal" group was plasma cortisol significantly and positively correlated with behavioral arousal (see Table 6.5). Higher cortisol

TABLE 6.4
Obstetrical and Physical Characteristics

	"Optimal"	*"NonOptimal"*
Birthweight		
<3000 grms	0	12
>4000 grms	0	3
Gestational Age		
36–47 wks	0	4
42+wks	0	4
Emergency C-Section	0	7
5-min Apgar < 7	0	4

Note: Some "nonoptimal" newborns presented several signs. Littman and Parmalee index differed significantly $t(33) = 4.15$, $p < .01$ (from Gunnar, Isensee, & Fust, 1987).

TABLE 6.5
Plasma Cortisol and Brazelton Arousal Items

Arousal Items	*Optimal*	*Non-Optimal*
	$n = 35$	$n = 25$
Peak of excitement	−.14	.39**
Rapidity of build-up	.19	.40**
Irritability	.22	.40**
Activity	.17	.14
Liability of states	.04	.05
Tremulousness	−.10	.38*
Sum of Above	.10	.50***

Note: From Gunnar, Isensee, and Fust (1987).
$^{*}p < .10$
$^{**}p < .05$
$^{***}p < .01$

levels for the extremely healthy group were correlated with better or more active attempts at behavioral state regulation ($r = 0.35$ vs. $r = 0.19$ for the optimal and nonoptimal newborns, respectively). Thus, these data suggest that the pattern of relations between adrenocortical activity and behavior in the newborn not only depend on the nature of the stimulation, but also on the newborns' medical or health status. The Brazelton Exam, like weighing and measuring or a discharge exam, elicited self-calming, quiescent behavior with higher cortisol levels in extremely healthy newborns. However, for "nonoptimal" newborns it elicited behavioral distress at higher cortisol levels.

It is impossible to reconcile these data with the view that the adrenocortical system is triggered by emotional or behavioral arousal. But if it is not a measure of emotional arousal, what kind of a model can encompass the results obtained in our own data and the data of others? This question must really be posed in two parts: (a) How can we characterize the events which trigger activation of the adrenocortical system, and (b) How can we model the relations between adrenocortical activity and behavior? In the following section we try to deal with the first question.

THE ADRENOCORTICAL SYSTEM AND CHANGING DEMANDS

In recent reviews of cortisol as a measure of stress, the importance of novelty, unpredictability, and strangeness have received increased attention (Levine, 1985; Rose, 1980). In one review, Rose (1980) noted that "it is apparent that individuals show a significant adrenal cortical activation when exposed to important *changes* in their environment" (p. 254, italics added). Furthermore, echoing Mason's (1975) earlier conclusion, Rose argued that the stressful psychological stimuli shown to elicit neuroendocrine responses are "acute or novel in nature, and that upon reexposure, endocrine responses extinguish." He supported this latter point with data on the adrenocortical system, contrasting the rapid extinction in response of this system with the continued response of the sympathetic-adrenomedullary system. Rose, however, stopped short of concluding that activation of the adrenocortical system was independent of systems regulating emotional distress. Indeed, he stated that both distress and novelty play a role in its regulation (p. 251). In contrast, Levine (1985) has specifically stated that cortisol is not "the emotion juice." Instead, he has argued, uncertainty is the primary psychological trigger of the pituitary-adrenocortical system. Uncertainty as the result of lack of predictability, discrepancy, violation of expectancy, or strangeness is a collative variable and, therefore, should produce arousal according to Berlyne (1960). Levine's view that cortisol reflects uncertainty is thus in line with his earlier argument that we can index arousal through measuring activity of the adrenocortical system (Hennessy & Levine, 1979).

The perception of novelty, strangeness, or unpredictability requires some degree of cognitive processing. Although newborns are capable of higher cortical activity under some circumstances, to describe the responses we have observed as reactions to uncertainty would seem to be "too cognitive." Instead, in order to encompass the entire course of development, we suggest that the basic stimulus of this neuroendocrine system may be better described as "significant changes in demands that the organism is not immediately prepared to meet." These demands may arise internally or externally. In more mature organisms biased toward responding in accordance to cognitive appraisals of events, uncertainty may constitute a primary demand: a demand for increased cognitive processing. It should be noted that this description of the stimuli capable of modulating the adrenocortical response may be able to encompass both physical and psychological events. Physical stimuli such as cold, heat, blood volume loss, and insulin create changes in demands, and the magnitude of the adrenocortical response typically reflects not only the absolute change, but also the rate of change (Gann, Dallman, & Engeland, 1981). Even large changes in these physical parameters tend to elicit only a slight response if they occur gradually. Changes that occur gradually, of course, permit the organism to gradually prepare to meet the increased demand thus creating less of a discrepancy between the demand and the mobilization of resources necessary to accommodate the demand.

The literature on activation of the adrenocortical system is replete with evidence that individuals differ in their response to similar situations. A focus on changing demands, however, does allow for such differences. Individuals may differ in what they perceive as a change and in what constitutes a demand.

Furthermore, in line with theories of stress and coping (e.g., Lazarus, 1966), how the individual responds should be a function of the individual's coping resources: As noted, the perceived magnitude of the demand should depend on the individual's preparation to meet the demand. In addition, this hypothesis also encompasses evidence that the adrenocortical system can respond bidirectionally. For example, in what Levine has called his "whoopee" effect, suddenly increasing the food available to weight-restricted rats has been shown to lower corticosterone levels (Levine, Goldman, & Coover, 1972). A sudden increase in food, of course, constitutes a sudden decrease in demands, and thus would be expected to dampen activity in the hypothalamic-pituitary-adrenocortical axis. Finally, this view allows for a rapid return to baseline activity even under circumstances that produce prolonged or chronic behavioral and emotional arousal. Prolonged or chronic demands do not constitute, by definition, a change in demands and thus should not produce elevations in corticoids. It should be noted that it is not clear that this model can encompass the chronic elevations in corticoids reported in clinical depression.

Glucocorticoids and Coping

To argue that changes in demands play a major role in adrenocortical regulation frees us to consider ways in which behavior and emotion interact with this system without the problem of needing to explain away dissociations. Two individuals may experience a change as involving a similar increase in demands, and yet may respond emotionally in different ways. Similarly, both behavioral quiescence and behavioral activity would seem to be reasonable responses to changed demands depending on the circumstances and the particular demands imposed. However, stated bluntly, if adrenocortical activity does not index emotion or arousal why should psychologists bother to obtain measures of glucocorticoids? The answer is that the adrenocortical system serves important functions in the organism's adaptation to changing internal and external demands and that through understanding its interaction with emotional, behavioral, and cognitive systems we can obtain a more accurate and complete understanding of how we have evolved to cope with changing circumstances.

However, the question of what role the pituitary-adrenocortical system plays in the coping process is perplexing. The most frequent answer to this question is that through acting in a coordinated fashion with glucagon, growth hormone, and insulin, corticoids increase glucose availability and thus are part of the energy mobilization, "protective" response to stressful events. But if corticoids primarily serve this function, why the rapid return to baseline in prolonged or chronically stressful situations when energy would seem to be at least as necessary a coping requirement? Furthermore, corticoids have ubiquitous effects on organs and tissues, many of these effects having little to do with energy mobilization. Indeed, many of these effects do not appear to "protect" the organism from the negative effects of changing demands; quite the opposite. They are effects that lower the organism's ability to manage demands, in part, through dampening activity of the immunosystem (Borysenko, 1984).

Munck and his colleagues (1984) have recently provided an alternative to the "energy mobilization" answer to the question of what function the adrenocortical system serves in adaptation. They argue that corticoids are elevated in response to "stressful" events primarily because the processes they set in motion operate as antagonists to other stress-sensitive peripheral systems, helping to return the organism to a prestress state. The primary function, then, is to "turn down" or "turn off" the mobilization that occurs in reaction to increased demands. For the most part, these dampening effects take hours or days to develop and thus are often observed after corticoid levels have returned to baseline. Accordingly, only relatively brief elevations in corticoids at the onset of stressful stimulation would be necessary for this system to participate in more prolonged adaptations to altered environmental or psychological demands.

In articulating their viewpoint, Munck and his colleagues (1984) concentrated on the effects of glucocorticoids on peripheral organs and tissues. They did not address effects on the brain. Activity of the adrenocortical system does have effects on the central nervous system, and these effects emerge more rapidly than the dampening effects on the periphery. Broadly speaking, ACTH appears to have a stimulatory effect on central processes, whereas glucocorticoids have an inhibitatory effect (de Kloet & de Wied, 1980). Together, the changing levels of ACTH and corticoids appear to enhance the individual's ability to establish new responses to altered environmental demands (Henry, 1980).

In summary, the adrenocortical system may serve two crucial functions in the organism's adaptation to increased demands. Initially, glucocorticoids participate in energy mobilization, however, their primary function in interaction with ACTH during this initial phase may be to facilitate learning and behavioral adaptation. During the second phase, as hypothesized by Munck and his co-workers (1984), the primary function may be to dampen the activity of "stress"-sensitive peripheral systems. This latter function is served through processes set in motion by the initial release of glucocorticoids. Eventually, dampening effects are observed, but often after corticoid levels have returned to base.

CORTICOIDS-BEHAVIOR RELATIONS

Thus far we have dealt with the questions of what triggers the adrenocortical system and what role this neuroendocrine system plays in the organism's ability to cope with changed demands. We have not yet dealt with the question of how changes in adrenocortical activity may be related to behavior. This is a more difficult question and one best approached from a systems perspective (see Sameroff, 1983, for review). Biological organisms can be viewed as open systems; systems that, although containing numerous components (some of which are also systems) function as whole, single, integrated entities. One of the primary characteristics of a system is its capacity to compensate for, correct, or damp out the disturbing effects of the surround. Compensation results from the activation of multiple self-righting processes that operate to counteract both the immediate effects of the disturbing event and the effects of responding to the disturbance. The relations between adrenocortical activity and behavior must be viewed from the perspective of these self-righting processes.

There is no one necessary behavioral response to a sudden change in demands, and thus no one necessary type of behavior that should co-occur with elevations in circulating corticoids. The behavior exhibited by the organism must, at the least, depend on the species, developmental level, and the nature of the change in demands. In addition, individual differences mediate the response as they impact the organism's perception of the event and the organism's coping resources, both internal and external. The behavioral self-righting response, thus, should be relatively finely tuned to the specific stimulus experienced in the context of the organism's history, current status, and available resources. Given this analysis, what relations might be expected between behavioral self-righting or coping responses and elevations in circulating glucocorticoids?

The answer may be that the magnitude of the adrenal response is related not to a particular type of behavioral reaction but to the intensity with which behavioral self-righting processes are set into motion. Thus, if the behavioral self-righting process in the particular context involves signalling distress, individuals experiencing higher elevations in corticoids would be expected to exhibit the greatest or most intense expressions of distress. If, however, the behavioral self-righting process involves information seeking, those individuals experiencing the greatest elevations in corticoids would be expected to engage in the greatest or most intense attempts to seek information. In summary, the magnitude of the adrenocortical response should be related to the intensity of whatever coping process is initiated.

However, this analysis is probably only accurate during the early part of the first phase of responding to sudden changes in demands when behavioral and physiological responses are being set into motion. Once the various self-righting processes have been activated it is reasonable to expect that they will begin to interact. Elevations in ACTH and glucocorticoids may begin to influence CNS activity, which in turn may alter behavioral responding; behavioral responses may alter the adrenocortical system through either (a) changing actual or perceived demands (e.g., activation or active attempts to control the environment or of cognitive processes focused on altering the perception of the demand), or (b) the individual's capacity to respond to stimulation (e.g., withdrawing into sleep). Both the intensity relations during the early part of the first phase and the potential for interaction during the later part of this phase of response can be illustrated by reference to our data on human newborns.

Neonatal Data Revisited

The point that elevations in cortisol should be related to the intensity and not the type of behavioral coping response has already been illustrated in the pattern of correlations presented earlier. However, the use of the Pearson correlation coefficient assumes that there is a continuous dimension of behavioral arousal, and as importantly, that biologically significant elevations in cortisol occur in linear increments reflected through measures of total cortisol production. Both assumptions can be questioned (see Prechtl & O'Brien, 1982, regarding behavioral arousal). Because cortisol, like other steroid hormones, binds to protein (primarily cortisol-binding globulin: CBG), most of the cortisol in circulation is bound, and thus biologically inactive.[1] In addition to affinity, the percent of free to bound cortisol depends on the availabilaity of binding sites relative to the amount of cortisol in circulation. As cortisol levels increase, available binding sites decrease, until at some point the available binding sites become filled and free cortisol begins to increase much more rapidly. Thus, at some point in the adrenocortical response there is a quantitative shift in the increment of biologically active cortisol in relation to additional increments in the production of the hormone by the adrenal cortex. Relatively little attention has been paid to this shift in research on the psychobiology of this system. It seems reasonable to argue that elevations in plasma cortisol to levels below this "shift" constitute relatively minor variations in adrenocortical activity, whereas elevations to levels above this "shift" point are of greater biological significance. Furthermore, it would seem reasonable to expect that the activation of intense behavioral coping processes should be primarily associated with cortisol levels that begin to exceed available binding sites.

In our research we have used salivary measures of cortisol to assess the free, unbound fraction of the hormone and plasma measures to assess the combination of bound and free fractions (Riad-Fahmy, Read, Joyce, & Walker, 1981). Human neonates exhibit relatively low plasma cortisol levels, yet the percentage of free hormone is much higher than that of older children and adults because of low levels of CBG (Hadjian, Chedin, Cochet, & Chambaz, 1975). For example, using 22 healthy newborns sampled randomly in the nursery we have found averaged plasma cortisol levels of 5 μg/dl associated with average salivary cortisol levels of 0.86 μg/dl.[2] Although one cannot convert from salivary to

[1]There is some disagreement over whether bound cortisol serves a biologically active function in certain organs and metabolic processes (see Riad-Fahmy, Read, & Hughes, 1979).

[2]In sampling saliva in infants we have collected the saliva on cotton dental rolls. We have found that some vegetable steroid in the cotton cross-reacts with our RIA assay resulting in a reading of between 0.03 and 0.05 μg/dl higher than actual.

plasma levels or vice versa (see Peters, Walker, Riad-Fahmy, & Hall, 1982), these salivary concentrations are sevenfold to eightfold higher than those reported with similar plasma concentrations in older children (Burke et al., 1985) and adults (Turkes, Morton, & Griffiths, 1985) and are comparable to salivary concentrations in neonates reported by others (e.g., 0.72 μg/dl; Price, Close, & Fielding, 1983). In adults the binding capacity of CBG under normal circumstances approximates 20 μg/dl (Riad-Fahmy, Read, & Hughes, 1979); the capacity in the neonate should be much lower.

To examine the relation between free and total cortisol we obtained paired salivary and plasma samples from 97 newborns under a variety of conditions including resting undisturbed, 20 minutes after a discharge exam, and heel-stick blood sampling. In each case, the salivary sample was obtained first (within 10 minutes of disturbance) and the heel-stick blood sample was taken immediately thereafter. To examine the absolute relations between salivary and plasma cortisol we grouped the plasma values into 5-point increments and averaged across salivary values obtained within these groupings. The resuls are shown in Fig. 6.4. As can be seen, the increment in salivary concentrations relative to plasma concentrations is relatively linear between the 1–5, 6–10, and 11–15 μg/dl groupings; however, at 16+μg/dl of plasma cortisol, salivary cortisol concentrations elevate precipitiously. Taking into account potential individual

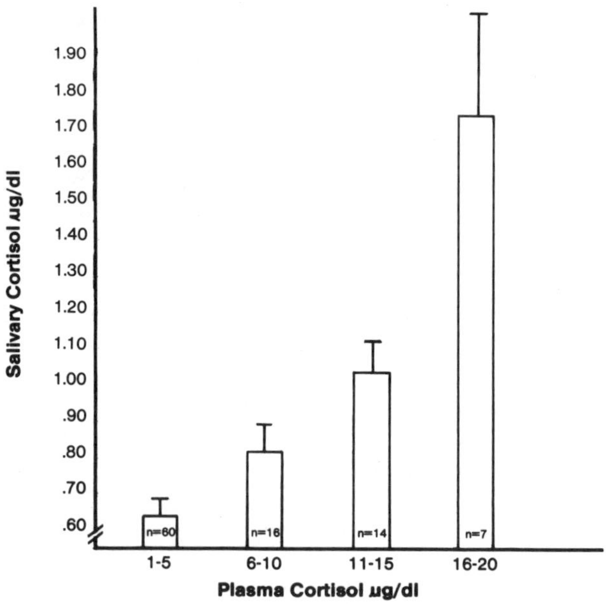

FIG. 6.4. Average salivary cortisol for 5 μg/dl groupings of plasma cortisol in human newborns (unpublished data). Bars represent SEM.

differences, the "shift" in free to total cortisol appears to occur somewhere around 16 μg/dl plasma (bound plus free) concentrations. It is at this point that, on the average, it would seem reasonable to describe the neonatal adrenocortical response as a "stress" reaction, and at this point, then, that we could expect to see a clear expression of behavioral coping reactions.

This is illustrated in the following figures (see Fig. 6.5, 6.6, 6.7). The first figure shows average behavioral state grouped again by 5-point increments in plasma cortisol concentrations using data from the study of responses to heel-stick blood sampling, weighing and measuring and the discharge exam described earlier (Gunnar, 1986b; Gunnar, Wall, & DeBoer, 1985). The difference between behavioral responses to heel–stick blood sampling and the weigh and measure or discharge exam are slight until plasma levels of cortisol exceed 16 μg/dl. Then the behavioral responses to these different events diverge sharply, with the newborns in the heel-stick condition fussing and crying and the newborns in the other two conditions withdrawing into a sleepy, drowsy state. These different behavioral reactions observed in conjunction with high plasma cortisol levels can now be seen as active coping responses that differ with

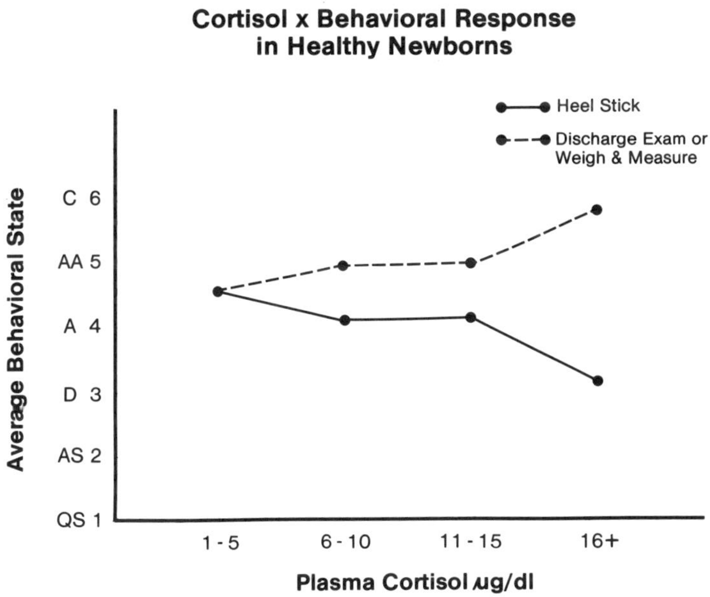

FIG. 6.5. Behavioral responses averaged for 5 μg/dl groupings of plasma cortisol obtained 20 min after the onset of either heel-stick blood sampling, weighing and measuring or a discharge-exam. Data collapsed across groups reported on in Gunnar, Connors, Isensee, and Wall (1988) and Gunnar (1986b).

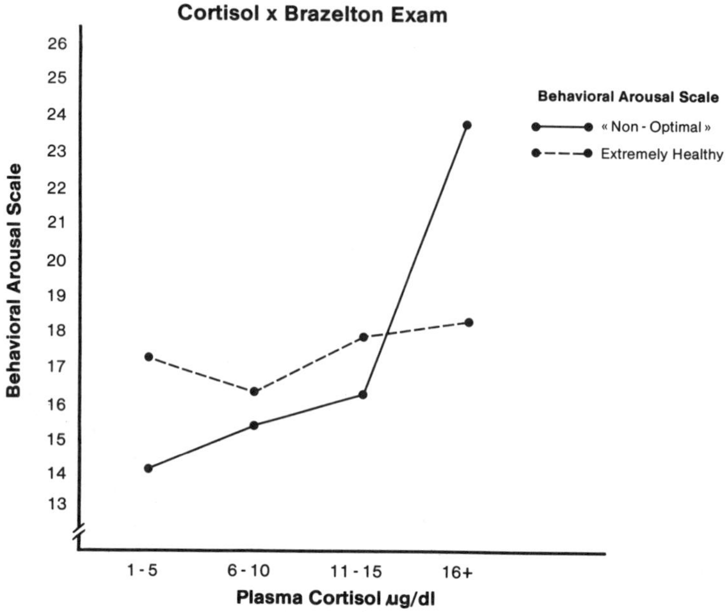

FIG. 6.6. Behavioral arousal scored by 5 μg/dl groupings of plasma cortisol in response to the Brazelton Neonatal Assessment Scale exam (derived from data reported in Gunnar, Isensee, & Fust, 1987).

the type of eliciting stimulus: Painful stimuli are associated with crying, which should bring aid from caregivers; nonpainful stimuli are associated with drowsiness and withdrawal that should reduce the newborn's responsiveness to stimulation. This latter reaction has been referred to as the "raising of a stimulus barrier," a behavioral strategy often described as one of the newborn's primary means of coping with disturbing events (Emde, Harmon, Metcalf, Koenig, & Wagonfeld, 1971).

However, as noted earlier, whether the newborn withdraws or cries may not only depend on the type of stimulation but also the newborn's biomedical status. Newborn's with more nonoptimal signs may not be able to readily tolerate even intense, nonnoxious stimulation and may respond with behavioral distress. Regardless, the triggering of the behavioral coping response should be most apparent for newborns responding with high cortisol levels. In Fig. 6.6 we see this pattern comparing behavioral arousal/distress for extremely healthy and "nonoptimal" newborns in response to the Brazelton exam (Gunnar, Isensee, & Fust, 1987); responses diverge most sharply for newborns with cortisol levels at or above 16 μg/dl. In Fig. 6.7, data on behavioral quiescence/withdrawal are shown for the same newborns: here again the clearest evidence of divergence in

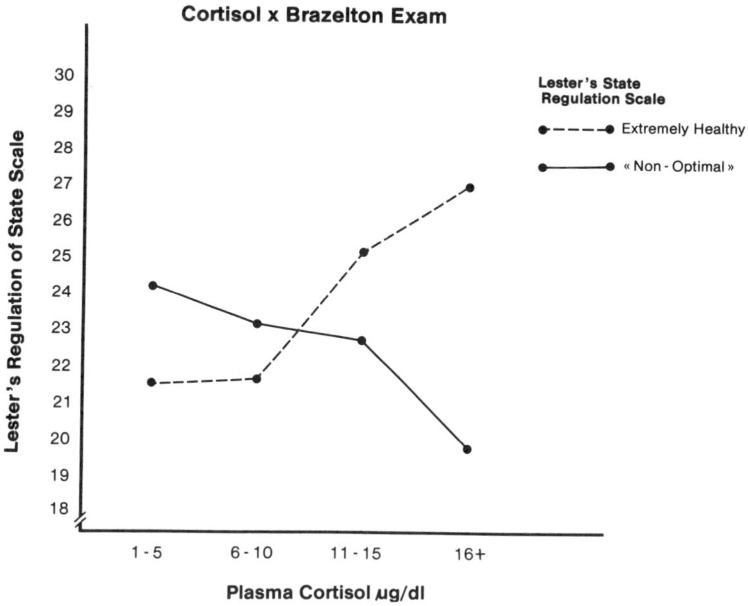

FIG. 6.7. Self-regulation scores by 5 μg/dl groupings of plasma cortisol in response to the Brazelton Neonatal Assessment Scale exam (derived from data reported in Gunnar, Isensee, & Fust, 1987).

behavioral response is seen for newborns with levels at or above 16 μg/dl. In summary, none of these data show a simple linear increase in some behavioral pattern associated with linear increments in total cortisol concentrations; instead, they show a "kicking in" of active, behavioral self-righting processes associated with stimulation eliciting high plasma cortisol levels.

The relations described earlier probably do not reflect either an effect of behavior on the adrenocortical system or an effect of cortisol on the CNS and thus on behavior. This is because the plasma cortisol measures were obtained after the behavioral measures, thus the behavioral measures were obtained while plasma cortisol was still rising and before levels had achieved peak elevations. The most likely period for observing interactions between cortisol and behavior would be in the hours following the initial activation of both systems. Furthermore, in the newborn the most probable interaction would be one of cortisol producing a reduction in behavioral activity that would, in turn, serve to reduce the newborn's adrenocortical responsiveness to stimulation thus facilitating the return of cortisol levels to baseline. An inhibitory effect of adrenocortical activation is predicted based on the fact that high levels of free cortisol should have a tonic, sedative effect on the CNS. In newborns, high concentrations of free cortisol are achieved at relatively low plasma cortisol concentrations as noted earlier.

We obtained data suggestive of this hormone-behavior interaction in a study of routine neonatal circumcision in which we examined behavior and plasma cortisol levels during the first four hours following circumcision (Gunnar, Malone, Vance, & Fisch, 1985). As in an earlier report by Emde and his colleagues (1971), following circumcision we observed an increase in the percentage of time spent in quiet, nonREM sleep (see Fig. 6.8). This increment in nonREM sleep followed extremely high levels of plasma cortisol produced in response to a combination of blood sampling and circumcision. This may reflect a sedative effect of stress levels of unbound cortisol. Furthermore, the greatest increment in quiet, nonREM sleep was noted during the period when plasma cortisol levels were decreasing most rapidly. Following perturbations such as circumcision, the increase in quiet sleep may help dampen the responsiveness of the adrenocortical system to stimulation, reduce any further production of cortisol, and thus facilitate the process of clearing cortisol from circulation.

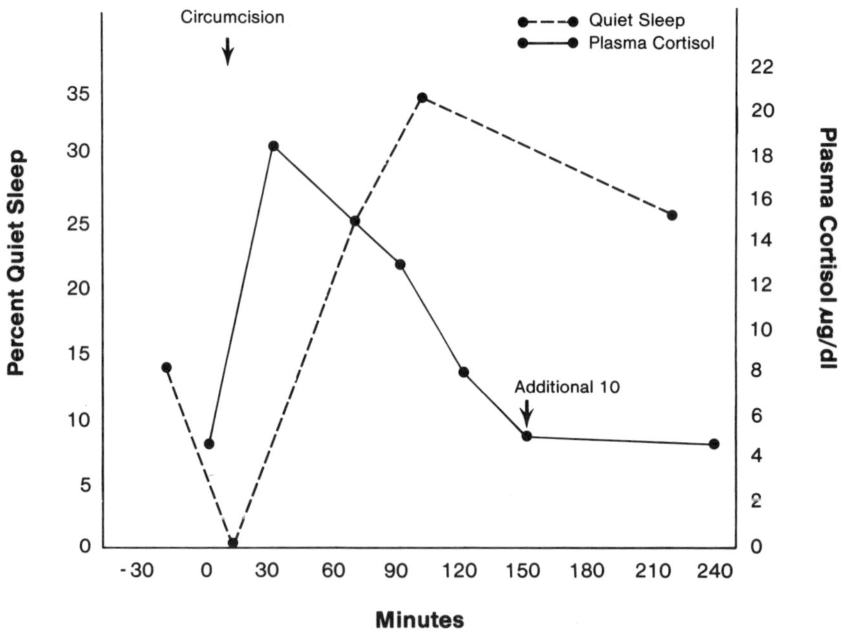

FIG. 6.8. Plasma cortisol and quiet sleep in newborns before, during and following circumcision. Additional 10 subjects studied at 150 min to determine time of return to baseline (derived from data reported in Gunnar, Malone, Vance, & Fisch, 1985).

HORMONE-COGNITION-BEHAVIOR RELATIONS

The sedative effects of increased adrenocortical activity should begin to decrease over the first year of life as CBG concentrations increase, and thus as higher concentrations of ACTH (CNS-stimulatory) are required to produce high concentrations of unboud cortisol (CNS-inhibitory). Therefore, with development the primary initial effect of the activation of the adrenocortical system should be the cognitive effect of facilitating the establishment of new behavioral patterns. Furthermore, as the child's cognitive abilities develop, uncertainty (novelty, unpredictability, strangeness) should become a primary trigger of this neuroendocrine system.

However, uncertainty is an extremely global variable. Should we expect that any experience of uncertainty will trigger elevations in glucocorticoids, or is only a certain type or degree of uncertainty capable of activating the pituitary-adrenocortical system? The answer may be that, uncertainty only triggers the adrenocortical system when it plays a role in increasing the demands the individual experiences. This is most likely to occur when uncertainty centers on the individual's self-efficacy expectancies (Bandura, 1977). Under such conditions uncertainty should stimulate an intense search for information and the mobilization of a variety of behavioral responses in the service of finding a response which might be effective. It is the search for information and the mobilization in service of establishing effective coping strategies which should constitute the increase in demands capable of triggering elevations in corticoids in response to self-efficacy uncertainty. A similar conclusion was reached by Weinberg and Levine (1980) in a review of the effects of predictability on activation of the adrenocortical system. In addition, this argument is consistent with Weiss' (1971) data on the importance of signalling the efficacy of a coping response in determining whether controlling the occurrence of an aversive event increases or decreases the adrenocortical response. Finally, this argument is also consistent with data on the effects of lack and loss of control on elevations in glucocorticoids (Hanson, Larson, & Snowdon, 1976).

A focus on self-efficacy uncertainty is particularly relevant to a developmental analysis of the role of uncertainty in regulating activation of the adrenocortical system. By the latter part of the first year, children have developed the cognitive capacity to experience uncertainty in novel situations and in response to unfamiliar people and events (Bronson, 1971). However, it is unlikely that infants and young children experience elevations in glucocorticoids in response to every uncertain encounter (Lundberg, 1983). Indeed, according to this analysis, this should occur only under conditions in which the infant or young child is uncertain about his or her ability to cope effectively with the demands arising in novel, unpredictable, or strange environments.

Early in development, children's coping strategies are largely organized around the presence and availability of attachment figures (Bowlby, 1969). Loss or lack of the attachment figure should, thus, create the primary conditions for self-efficacy uncertainty early in development. Among the young of infrahuman primates this has been repeatedly demonstrated. Separation from the mother triggers significant elevations in cortisol; the presence of alternate caregivers facilitates a rapid reduction in elevated levels; the presence of the mother can prevent an adrenocortical response even to seemingly drastic alterations in the environment (Coe & Levine, 1981; Gunnar, Gonzales, Goodlin, & Levine, 1981a). The only related study with human children was conducted by Tennes and Vernadakis (1977). Using urinary measures of corticoid metabolites, they failed to observe elevations among separated 12-month-olds. However, the presence of warm, supportive alternate caregivers in the Tennes and Vernadakis study may have served to help the infants cope, reduce their uncertainty, and thus prevent an adrenocortical response to separation.

Developmental Factors

Among adults, uncertainty over one's ability to manage the demands of situations may reflect individual differences in efficacy beliefs or variations among situations and individuals in the availability of coping resources. Among children, however, such uncertainty may also arise as the result of developmental changes which alter the child's understanding of situations and of the behaviors which constitute "effective" coping. We first became sensitive to the importance of self-efficacy uncertainty in the context of studying the relations between behavioral distress and adrenocortical activity among children with phenylketonuria (PKU). We were studying these children during clinic visits that involved blood sampling (Marvinney, Isensee, Fisch, & Gunnar, 1986 unpublished manuscript). Our interest in this group of children was three-fold. First, this group had been identified at birth, had been treated in the same clinic by the same doctor since early infancy, and during each clinic visit experienced the same routine that culminated in the doctor taking a blood sample either from the scalp (infant) or arm (toddlers and older children). By studying this group of children we hoped to be able to examine the relations between behavioral distress and adrenocortical activity without what we then viewed as the confounding effect of novelty. Second, because these children had been treated since birth, their intellectual growth was relatively normal. In addition, we eliminated from our sample children whose DQ or IQ was below normal. Although these childrlen constituted a group who had to undergo aversive medical procedures frequently, they were nonetheless a relatively normal, healthy group of children from our perspective. Third, the clinic staff enticed us into conducting this study with their descriptions of developmental changes in behavioral distress. They reported that preschool children were typically the most distressed in the clinic relative to infants and older childrlen. If true, we hoped to demonstrate a developmental change in adrenocortical activation to the clinic visit which corresponded to the developmental change in behavioral distress.

In a first study we simply had an observer and the physician independently rate the children on a scale of emotional distress and we had the parent record whether the child was distressed, acting normally or acting subdued during different phases of the clinic visit (waiting room, physical exam, blood draw, and so on). These measures were found to be highly intercorrelated (r' s = > .80). In addition, we took blood for plasma cortisol determination when the sample was drawn for assessment of pherylalanine level. As shown in Fig. 6.9, we did see a significant change in behavioral distress with age with the preschoolers being the most distressed. Counter to expectations, however, the pattern for cortisol was offset from that of behavioral distress. It looked as if cortisol production increased during the older developmental period, when the children were becoming less distressed or perhaps learning to inhibit expressions of their distress in the clinic.

Learning to act grown up is terribly important for children during the late preschool, early elementary school years. This is also the time when children are beginning to learn rules about the situational determinants of emotions they can

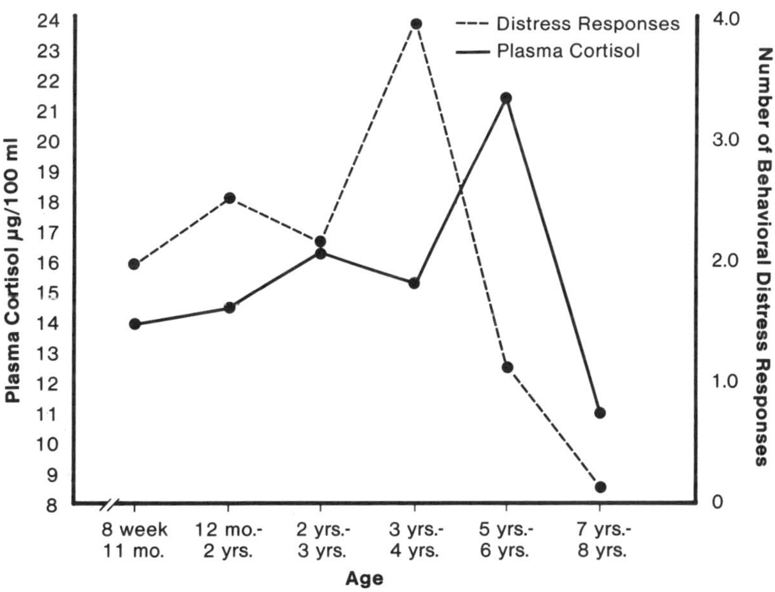

FIG. 6.9. Behavioral distress and plasma cortisol during clinic visits in children with PKU (Marvinney, Isensee, Fisch, & Gunnar, 1986).

and should display (Saarni, 1979), and they are coming to understand that emotions are internal events that can be regulated by internal processes (Carroll & Steward, 1984). However, their understanding of emotions and emotion regulation is far from complete, thus their ability to regulate their own emotional displays is far from certain. We began to suspect that what appeared to be an elevation in cortisol during the late preschool years in these data was an expression of the children's uncertainty about whether they would be successful in inhibiting their distress, so as not to appear to be "acting like a baby."

To examine this hypothesis, we completed a second study in which we obtained a plasma cortisol as before from 23 children between 3 and 10 years of age (16 had been tested earlier). In addition, we managed to get home and clinic salivary cortisol estimates on 10 children, which allowed us to derive upper and lower limits of baseline levels for these children during the morning clinic hours. We also conducted interviews with the children following the clinic visit. The interview questions were designed to tap the child's understanding of emotions and, as shown in Table 6.6, responses to these questions were highly correlated with age, although not with IQ in this small sample. Interviews from 7 of the children had to be eliminated either because the child was too shy to answer the questions ($n = 3$), did not appear to understand the questions ($n = 1$), had an older sibling in the room who answered the questions for the child ($n = 1$), or refused to go with the interviewer or answer the questions ($n = 2$).

In this study we were interested in three questions. First, would the offset pattern of behavioral distress and plasma cortisol replicate? Second, would we find evidence suggesting that this pattern reflected developmental change as opposed merely to individual differences? And third, would the pattern for plasma cortisol be related to uncertainty regarding emotion regulation? With regard to this last question, we were expecting that children who were at a middle level of understanding emotions would be the ones experiencing the elevations in cortisol, because these children should be both highly motivated to control expressions of distress and highly uncertain about their ability to do so.

As shown in Fig. 6.10, the hormone-behavior pattern did replicate. The peaks for behavioral distress and plasma cortisol were, however, shifted slightly to the right, suggesting that individual differences were affecting what appeared to be a pattern of developmental change. This was also supported by the correlations for both behavioral distress [$r(14) = 0.74$, $p < .01$] and plasma cortisol [$r(14) = 0.61$, $p < .05$] for the children whom we had tested in both studies. However, as shown in Fig. 6.11, a plot of the plasma cortisol data from both studies continued to reveal the pattern of initial decline as children moved into the preschool period, followed by a rise in the late preschool period, followed by a decline among the older children. These data indicate that both individual differences and developmental change were contributing to the hormonal pattern.

Finally, as shown in Fig. 6.12, children who received mid-range scores on the

TABLE 6.6
Emotion Understanding Scale

	Correlations Item-total
1. Why do children cry in the clinic?	.57
0 = No idea	
1 = External (get a shot)	
2 = Physical (it hurts)	
3 = Feeling (scared)	
2. How can you change or hide upset feelings?	.77
0 = No idea	
1 = External (Adult stop crying)	
2 = Change Own (Just stop)	
3 = Self-initiated strategies (thoughts)	
3. If a child does not cry or look upset on the outside while blood is drawn, how does the child feel on the inside?	.64
0 = no idea	
1 = happy (outside and inside consistent)	
2 = sad (hide emotion)	
3 = mixed (multiple feelings)	
4. Are multiple feelings possible?	.80
0 = no idea	
1 = sequential	
2 = simultaneous	
5. How do you feel when your blood is tested?	.63
0 = no response	
1 = one emotion (happy or sad)	
2 = mixed emotion (happy and sad)	
6. Why do you watch (not watch) your blood being drawn?	.35
0 = no idea	
1 = some explanation	
7. How many nonblood test thoughts did the child generate as "things to think about" while waiting for the blood test?	.38
0 = none	
1 = one or more ideas	

Total possible points = 15
Score was the percentage of possible points.
Correlation of scale scores with age was +.77.
Questions do not reflect actual phrasing of the interview questions.

emotion understanding interview were the ones who exhibited elevations in cortisol [test for curvilinearity using $(X\text{-}\overline{X})^2 = X_T$ was significant, $r(13) = -.56$, $p < .05$]. Qualitatively these children, compared to children receiving less than 40% of the total possible points, believed that children could look happy outside but be sad or scared inside, and they believed that adults could change children's emotions, but were not sure that children could. Furthermore, unlike the children receiving 60% or more of the total possible points, these children could

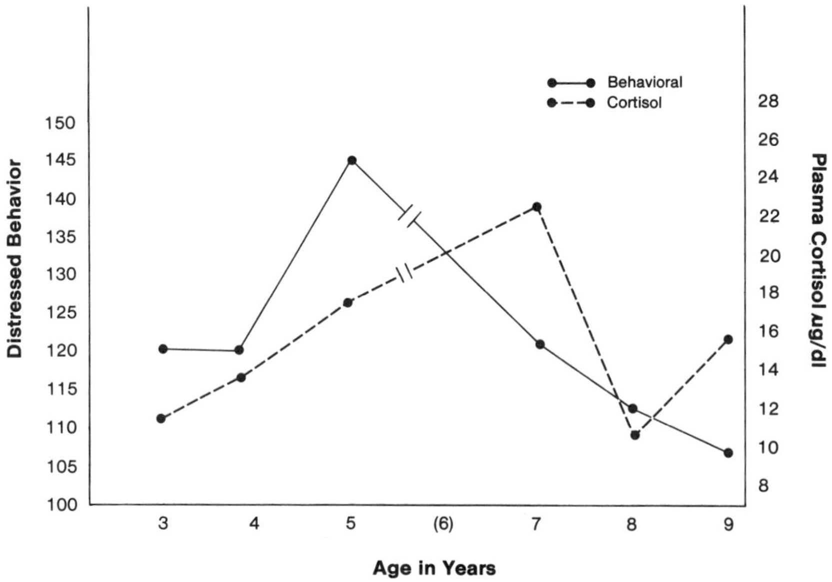

FIG. 6.10. Behavioral distress and plasma cortisol from follow-up study of children with PKU (Marvinney et al., 1986).

not elaborate strategies for controlling their own emotions. When asked how a child might stop crying, a typical mid-level response would be "he would just stop." A mid-level understanding of emotions combined with the desire to avoid acting like a baby would, thus, seem to be a prescripton for experiencing a significant degree of self-efficacy uncertainty.

These data indicate that situations need not be unfamiliar in order to elicit elevations in corticoids among children. They also point to the importance of a developmental analysis of children's responses to difficult situations. Indeed, they suggest that the process of development, encompassing as it does periods of transition during which children are actively reorganizing their responses to events in the service of achieving new, more mature standards for their behavior, may play a major role in the activation of the adrenocortical system. Finally, it is tempting to suggest that elevations in corticoids during these periods may not only reflect uncertainty regarding self-efficacy, but also aid in its resolution through facilitating the emergence of new behavior patterns.

SUMMARY

Activity of the adrenocortical system has been used inaccurately as an index of emotional distress and arousal. More recently, reviewers have emphasized the

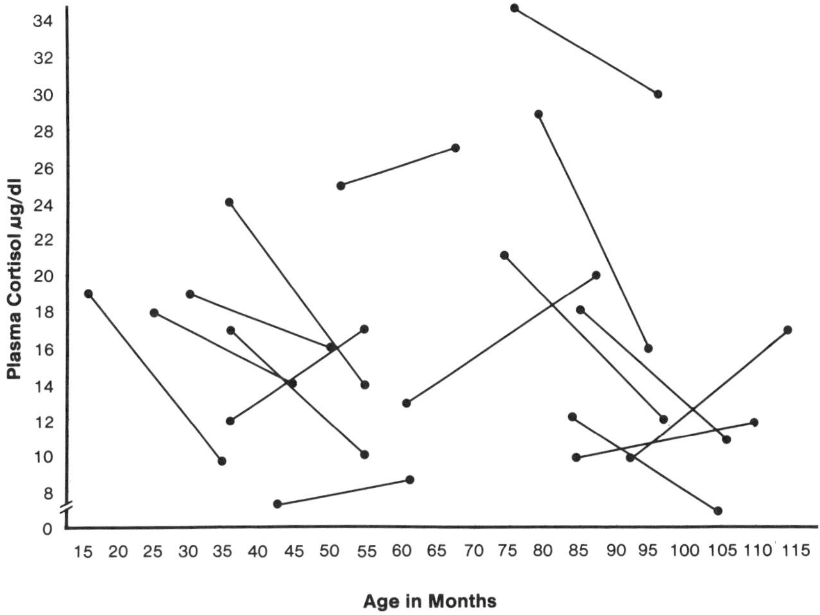

FIG. 6.11. Plasma cortisol for two clinic visits separated by an average of 20 months for 16 children with PKU (Marvinney et al. 1986).

importance of uncertainty in regulating this system. However, viewing uncertainty as the primary trigger of this neuroendocrine system is both too exclusive, in that it does not encompass the entire developmental spectrum, and too inclusive, in that it encompasses eliciting conditions that would not be expected to trigger elevations in glucocorticoids. Instead, it is proposed that the adrenocortical system is activated when the individual experiences a change in stimulation, involving an increase in demands, for which the individual does not have an immediately prepared response. The magnitude of the adrenocortical response should reflect the magnitude of the mobilization of resources required to meet the demand. With regard to uncertainty, in many instances cognitive uncertainty may merely be a correlate of the conditions necessary to trigger the adrenocortical response. Cognitive uncertainty is not expected to trigger elevations in cortisol unless it creates the conditions for further increases in demands relative to resources. This may occur most frequently when the relevant uncertainty involves self-efficacy expectations. Because efficacy standards change with development, situations that would seem to place similar demands on children may, in fact, place different demands on children who are at different levels of development. This latter point underscores the importance of maintaining a developmental perspective in

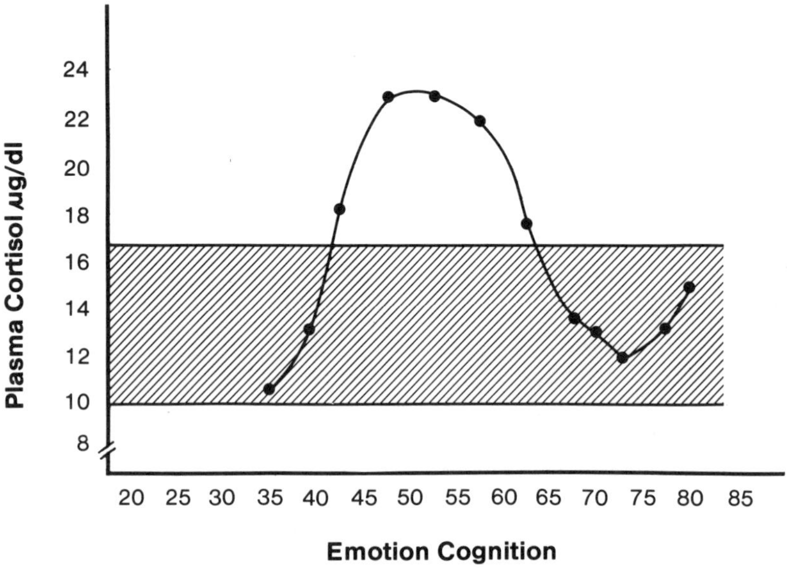

FIG. 6.12. Plasma cortisol as a function of emotion understanding. (Marvinney et al., 1986). (Graph produced using curve smoothing techniques. Analysis performed on raw data. Darkened area represents range for baseline cortisol.)

addressing the question of how children cope with challenging, demanding or difficult circumstances.

REFERENCES

Anders, T., Sachar, E., Kream, J., Roffwarg, H., & Hellman, L. (1970). Behavioral state and plasma cortisol response in the human newborn. *Pediatrics, 46*(4), 532–537.

Bandura, A. (1977). Self-efficacy: Towards a unifying theory of behavioral change. *Psychological Review, 84*, 191–215.

Berlyne, D. E. (1960). *Conflict, arousal and curiosity*. New York: McGraw-Hill.

Borysenko, J. (1984). Stress, coping, and the immune system. In J. D. Matarazzo, S. M. Weiss, J. A. Herd, & N. E. Miller (Eds.), *Behavioral health* (pp. 248–260). New York: Wiley.

Bowlby, J., (1969). *Attachment and Loss* (Vol. 1) *Attachment*. New York: Basic Books.

Brazelton, T. B. (1973). *Neonatal behavioral assessment scale* (Clinics in Developmental Assessment, No. 50). Philadelphia, PA: Lippincott.

Bronson, G. (1971). Fear of the unfamiliar in human infants. In H. R. Schaffer (Eds.), *Origins of human social relations* (pp. 59–71). New York: Academic Press.

Burke, P., Reichler, R., Smith, E., Dugaw, K., McCauley, E., & Mitchell, J. (1985). Correlation between serum and salivary cortisol levels in depressed and non-depressed children and adolescents. *American Journal of Psychiatry, 142*(9), 1065–1067.

Carroll, J., & Steward, M. S. (1984). The role of cognitive development in children's understanding of their own feelings. *Child Development, 55*, 1486–1492.

Coe, C. L., & Levine, S. (1981). Normal response to mother–infant separation in non-human primates. In D. F. Klein & J. Kaplan (Eds.), *Anxiety: New research and changing concepts* (pp. 155–177). New York: Raven Press.

de Kloet, R., & de Wied, D. (1980). The brain as target tissue for hormones of pituitary origin: Behavioral and biochemical studies. In L. Martini & W. F. Ganong (Eds.), *Frontiers in neuroendocrinology* (pp. 157–201). New York: Raven.

Emde, R. N., Harmon, R., Metcalf, D., Koenig, K., & Wagonfeld, S. (1971). Stress and neonatal sleep. *Psychosomatic Medicine, 33*, 491–497.

Feyerabend, P. K. (1970). Against method: Outline of an anarchistic theory of knowledge. In M. Radner & S. Winoker (Eds.), *Minnesota studies in the philosophy of science, Vol 4: Analysis of theories and methods in physics and psychology* (pp. 17–130). Minneapolis: University of Minnesota Press.

Frankenhaeuser, M. (1980). Psychobiological aspects of life stress. In S. Levine & H. Ursin (Eds.), *Coping and health* (pp. 203–224). New York: Plenum.

Gann, D. S., Dallman, M. F., & Engeland, W. E. (1981). Reflex control and modulation of ACTH and corticosteroids. In S. M. McCann (Ed.), *Endocrine physiology III: International review of physiology* (Vol. 24, pp. 157–194). Baltimore: University Park Press.

Gunnar, M. (1986a). Psychoneuroendocrine studies of stress and coping in human children. In M. Lamb, A. Brown, & B. Rogoff (Eds.), *Advances in developmental psychology* (Vol. 4, pp. 51–103). Hillsdale, NJ: Lawrence Erlbaum Associates.

Gunnar, M. (1986b, April). *The organization of stress responses in the newborn.* Paper presented at the International Conferences on Infant Studies, Los Angeles, CA.

Gunnar, M., Connors, J., Isensee, J., & Wall, L. (1988). Adrenocortical activity and behavioral distress in human newborns. *Developmental Psychobiology, 21*, 297–310.

Gunnar, M., Fisch, R., Korsvik, S., & Donhowe, J. (1981b). The effects of circumcision on serum cortisol and behavior. *Psychoneuroendocrinology*, 6(3), 269–276.

Gunnar, M., Fisch, R., & Malone, S. (1984). The effects of pacifying stimulus on behavioral and adrenocortical responses to circumcision. *Journal of the American Academy of Child Psychiatry, 23*, 34–38.

Gunnar, M., Gonzales, C., Goodlin, B., & Levine, S. (1981a). Behavioral and pituitary-adrenal responses during a prolonged separation period in infant rhesus macaques. *Psychoneuroendocrinology*, 6(1), 66–75.

Gunnar, M. Isensee, J., & Fust, S. (1987). Adrenocortical activity and the Brazelton neonatal assessment scale: Moderating effects of the newborn's biomedical status. *Child Development, 58*, 1448–1458.

Gunnar, M., Malone, S., Vance, G., & Fisch, R. (1985). Coping with aversive stimulation in the neonatal period: Quiet sleep and plasma cortisol during recovery from circumcision. *Child Development, 56*, 824–834.

Gunnar, M., Wall, L., & DeBoer, J. (1985, April). *A psychoendocrine study of stress versus distress in the human newborn.* Paper presented at the Society for Research and Child Developement, Toronto.

Hadjian, A. J., Chedin, M., Cochet, C., & Chambaz, E. M. (1975). Cortisol binding to proteins in plasma in the human neonate and infant. *Pediatric Research, 9*, 40–45.

Hanson, J. D., Larson, M. E., & Snowdon, C. T. (1976). The effects of control over high intensity noise on plasma cortisol levels in rhesus monkeys. *Behavioral Biology, 16,* 333–340.

Hennessy, J., & Levine, S. (1979). Stress, arousal and the pituitary-adrenal system: A psychoendocrine model. In J. Sprague & A. Epstein (Eds.), *Progress in psychobiological and physiological psychology* (Vol. 8, pp. 133–178). New York: Academic Press.

Henry, J. P. (1980). Present concept of stress theory. In E. Usdin, R. Kretnansky, & I. J. Kopin (Eds.), *Catecholamines and stress: Recent advances* (pp. 557–571). New York: Elsevier North Holland Inc.

Kuhn, T. S. (1970). *The structure of scientific revolutions* (2nd ed.). Chicago: University of Chicago Press.

Lazarus, R. S. (1966). *Psychological stress and the coping process.* New York: McGraw-Hill.

Levine, S. (1985). A definition of stress? In G. P. Moberg (Ed.), *Animal stress* (pp. 51–69). Bethesda, MD: American Physiological Society.

Levine, S., Goldman, L., & Coover, G. (1972). Expectancy and the pituitary-adrenal system. *Physiology, Emotion and Psychosomatic Illness.* (Ciba Foundation Symposium, 8, pp. 281–295). Amsterdam, North-Holland: Elsevier.

Lundberg, U. (1983). Sex differences in behavior pattern and catecholamine and cortisol excretion in 3–6 year old day-care childrlen. *Biological Psychology, 16,* 109–117.

Malone, S., Gunnar, M., & Fisch, R. (1985). Adrenocortical and behavioral responses to limb restraint and blood sampling in human neonates. *Developmental Psychobiology, 18*(5), 435–446.

Marvinney, D., Isensee, J., Fisch, R. O., & Gunnar, M. (1986). *Stress and distress among children with chronic illness,* unpublished manuscript.

Mason, J. W. (1959). Psychological influences on the pituitary-adrenal cortical system. In G. Pineus (Ed.), *Recent progress in hormone research* (Vol. 15, pp. 345–360). New York: Academic Press.

Mason, J. W. (1968). A review of psychoendoerine research on the pituitary-adrenal cortical system. *Psychosomatic Medicine, 30,* 576–608.

Mason, J. W. (1975). Emotions as reflected in patterns of endocrine integration. In L. Levi (Ed.), *Emotions—Their parameters and measurement* (pp. 143–181). New York: Raven Press.

Munck, A., Guyre, P., & Holbrook, N., (1984). Physiological functions of glucocorticoids in stress and their relations to pharmacological actions. *Endocrine Review, 5,* 25–43.

Peters, J. R., Walker, R., Riad-Fahmy, D., & Hall, R. (1982). Salivary cortisol assays for assessing pituitary–adrenal reserve. *Clinical Endocrinology, 17,* 583–592.

Popper, K. R. (1972). *Objective knowledge.* Oxford, England: Oxford University Press.

Prechtl, H., & O'Brien, M. J. (1982). Behavioral states of the full-term newborn: The emergence of a concept. In P. Stratton (Ed.), *Psychobiology of the human newborn.* (pp. 53–74). New York: Wiley.

Price, P. A., Close, G. C., & Fielding, B. A. (1983). Age of appearance of circadian rhythm in salivary cortisol values in infancy. *Archives of Diseases in Childhood, 58,* 454–456.

Riad-Fahmy, D., Read, G., & Hughes, I. A. (1979). Corticosteroids. In C. H. Gray & V. H. T. James (Eds.), *Hormones in blood* (Vol. 3, pp. 179–262). New York: Academic Press.

Riad-Fahmy, D., Read, G. F., Joyce, B. G., & Walker, R. F. (1981). Steroid immunoassays in endocrinology. In A. Vollar, A. Bartlett, & J. D. Bidwell (Eds.), *Immunoassays for the 80s* (pp. 205–261). Baltimore, MD: University Park Press.

Rose, R. M. (1980). Endocrine responses to stressful psychological events. Advances in psychoneuroendocrinology. *Psychiatric Clinics of North America, 3(2)*, 251–276.

Saarni, C. (1979). Children's understanding of display rules for expressive behavior. *Developmental Psychology, 15*, 424–429.

Sameroff, A. (1983). Developmental systems: Context and evolutions. In P. Mussen (Ed.), *Handbook of child psychology* (Vol. 1, pp. 237–294). New York: Wiley.

Tennes, K., & Carter, D. (1973). Plasma cortisol levels and behavioral states in early infancy. *Psychosomatic Medicine, 35*, 121–128.

Tennes, K., & Mason, J. (1982). Developmental psychoendocrinology: An approach to the study of emotions. In C. Izard (Ed.), *Measuring emotions in infants and children* (pp. 21–37). Cambridge, England: Cambridge University Press.

Tennes, K. & Vernadakis, A. (1977). Cortisol excretion levels and daytime sleep in one-year-old infants. *Journal of Clinical Endocrinology and Metabolism, 44*, 175–179.

Turkes, A., Morton, M. S., & Griffiths, K. (1985). The application of some newer aspects of immunoassay to clinical endocrinology. *Biochemical Society Transactions, 13*, 397–400.

Ursin, H., Baade, E., & Levine, S. (1978). *Psychobiology of stress.* New York: Academic Press.

Weinberg, J., & Levine, S. (1980). Psychobiology of coping in animals: The effects of predictability. In S. Levine & H. Ursin (Eds.), *Coping and health* (pp. 39–59). New York: Plenum Press.

Weiss, J. M. (1971). Effects of coping behavior with and without a feedback signal on stress pathology in rats. *Journal of Comparative Physiology and Psychology, 77*, 22–30.

Wolff, C. T., Hofer, M. A., & Mason, J. W. (1964). Relationship between psychological defenses and mean urinary 17–OHCS excretion rates: II. Methodological and theoretical considerations. *Psychosomatic Medicine, 26*, 592–609.

7

The Constructs of Inhibition and Lack of Inhibition to Unfamiliarity

Jerome Kagan
Nancy Snidman
Harvard University

J. Steven Reznick
Yale University

Most commentators on human nature have noted that the variation in the reaction to unfamiliarity and possible risk is a major characteristic that differentiates adults. Even though it is rare to find a large number of people who are consistently shy, cautious, and timid, or, on the other hand, outgoing, relaxed, and bold in all contexts, there is a small group, perhaps 10%, who consistently bring one or the other of these behavioral styles to untried situations that have the potential to create uncertainty. Jung's category of introversion–extraversion represents the most complete elaboration of this idea, and empirical indices of these and related constructs are among the most stable and the most heritable in contemporary psychological research (Conley, 1985; Loehlin, 1982; Plomin, 1986). The actualization of these two qualities in childhood has been described by Thomas and Chess (1977), who generated great interest among psychologists in the study of temperament.

The hypothesis that children differ in the ease with which inhibition of action and/or withdrawal are evoked by unfamiliarity and challenge is implicit in Sheldon's tripartite typology, as well as Schneirla's (1959, 1965) suggestion that approach or withdrawal from events is a fundamental differentiating feature in animal species. Moreover, the empirical record affirms this idea for many animal groups, including mice, rats, cats, dogs, wolves, pigs, and monkeys. Blizard (1981) found these strain differences among rats, Scott and Fuller (1974) discovered that timidity was one of the two most differentiating characteristics in five breeds of dogs, and Suomi (1984) as well as Stevenson-Hinde and her colleagues (1980) reported that variation in timid behavior was a stable quality in macaque monkeys reared in a laboratory from infancy to puberty.

In childhood, a temperamental quality defined by initial tendency to withdraw, to seek a parent, and to inhibit play and vocalization following encounter with unfamiliar people or events persists over the childhood years and is part of a coherent network of behavioral and physiological characteristics (Bronson, 1981; Kagan & Moss, 1962). This quality was the only one preserved from the first three years of life through childhood and adolescence in the Fels Research Institute's Longitudinal population (Kagan & Moss, 1962). A subsequent longitudinal study also found that among infants and young children from Caucasian and Chinese families living in the Boston area, behavioral timidity was the best preserved characteristic from 3 through 29 months of age (Kagan, Kearsley, & Zelazo, 1978). Follow-up investigations of clinical cases reveal modest preservation of extreme forms of withdrawal behavior from childhood to adult life. A group of 66 children diagnosed as school phobic when they were between 4 and 11 years of age were assessed by a psychiatrist when they were 12 to 21 years old. About 25% of the group had no symptoms and were regarded as well adjusted. Although another 40% were no longer phobic, they still displayed one or more other symptoms, especially poor school achievement and a sense of dependency on others. An additional 33% was still very anxious (Coolidge, Brodie, & Feeney, 1964). As might be expected, extremely shy, phobic children are likely as adults to select bureaucratic jobs with minimal risk (Morris, Soroker, & Burruss, 1954).

Although preservation of these two complementary classes of behavior does not require the assumption of biological factors, research implicates genetic influences. Studies of monozygotic and dyzygotic twins—infants, adolescents, and adults—reveal that the psychological characteristics yielding the best evidence of heritability are related to approach or withdrawal to the unfamiliar (see Plomin, 1986, for an extensive review of this literature). For example, examiners rated the test behavior of a large number of twins six times between 3 and 24 months of age. Factor analysis revealed a factor of timidity and inhibition that showed evidence of heritability at 6, 12, and 24 months of age (Matheny, 1980). In a similar investigation, behavioral ratings were made on 350 twin pairs at 8 months, 4 years, and 7 years (Goldsmith & Gottesman, 1981). Differences in fearfulness, indexed by reluctance to separate from the mother at 7 years of age, were among the most heritable of the behavioral variables, especially for boys. Finally, the heritabiliity of the social introversion score on the MMPI in adolescent twin pairs, which is often a developmental derivative of extreme withdrawal in childhood, was higher than any of the other MMPI scales, and again, the coefficients were higher for male than for female twins (Gottesman, 1963; see also, Eaves & Eysenck, 1975; Loehlin, 1982).

LONGITUDINAL STUDIES OF INHIBITION

Our laboratory has been studying two independent groups of Caucasian children from intact middle- and working-class families who were selected from larger samples when they were either 21 or 31 months of age because the child was either consistently shy, timid, and fearful (we call such children *behaviorally inhibited)* or sociable, bold, and fearless *(uninhibited)* when exposed to unfamiliar rooms, people, and objects. We had to screen over 400 children using both telephone interviews and laboratory observations in order to select groups of approximately 60 inhibited and 60 uninhibited children with equal numbers of boys and girls in each group (see Garcia-Coll, Kagan, & Reznick, 1984; Snidman, 1984; for details). It is of interest that when German kindergarten teachers in Munich were asked to select only those children who were extremely shy, only 15% of the total school population of 1,100 was chosen (Cranach et al., 1978).

The original index of inhibition in Cohort 1 at 21 months of age was based on behavior with an unfamiliar woman, unfamiliar toys, a woman displaying some acts that were somewhat difficult to recall and imitate, a metal robot, and temporary separation from the mother. The behaviors that were regarded as operational definitions of inhibition were long latencies to interact with or retreat from the unfamiliar people or objects, staying proximal to the mother, and cessation of play or vocalization. The index of inhibited behavior in the second cohort at 31 months of age was based primarily on behavior with an unfamiliar child of the same sex and age, and second on behavior with an unfamiliar woman. However, the definitions of inhibition were similar to those used with the first cohort, namely long latencies to interact with the child, adult, or toys, and long periods of time remaining proximal to the mother. Each of these groups has been seen several additional times since the original selection. Cohort 1 was seen again at 4, 5½ years, and 7½years. Cohort 2 was seen at 43 months, 5½years, and is currently being evaluated at 7½years of age (see Kagan et al., 1984; Kagan, Reznick, & Snidman, in press; Reznick et al., 1986; Snidman, 1984, for additional details.)

PRESERVATION OF BEHAVIOR

The behaviors that characterize the two classes of children were preserved from the original to the later assessments. For example, for Cohort 1 the correlation between an aggregate index of inhibition at 21 months and an aggregate index at 5½years was $+.52$ ($p < .001$). For Cohort 2, the correlation between the aggregate index of inhibited behavior at 31 months and the index at 5½years was .55 ($p < .01$).

One of the most sensitive indexes of this quality in school-age children is a group play session with 8 to 10 unfamiliar children of the same sex. This evaluation was implemented with Cohort 1 when they were 7½ years of age. The 90-minute session consisted of free-play intervals interspersed with supervised competitive games. The videotaped records of the sessions, supplemented by taped narrations of each child's behavior by observers who did not know the child's prior history, were coded for several variables. The two most sensitive were: total time each child was distant from and not interacting with another child during free-play intervals (defined as greater than an arm's length from any other child), and number of spontaneous utterances. This index of inhibition, based on the mean standard score for these two variables, was related to the earlier indexes of inhibition ($r = 0.6$). However, the coefficients do not capture the consistency with which a majority of inhibited children habitually moved away from other children. When the group was lined up for a game, it was most often the inhibited child who was at the far end of the line or standing a few feet in back of the group. When a child approached a formerly inhibited child the latter would often walk away within a few seconds. Throughout the 90-minute session it was the inhibited children who would typically move away from wherever the center of the group was located, especially when the children at the center were engaged in rough and tumble play. It was as if a small cluster of unfamiliar childrlen constituted an aversive object to be avoided. These observations remind us of Jung's (1924) definitions of his two basic psychological types:

> Extraversion means the outward turning of the libido . . . a positive movement of subjective interests towards the object (p. 542). . . . Introversion means a turning inwards of the libido whereby a negative relation of subject to object is expressed. Interest does not move towards the object, but recedes towards the subject. (p. 567)

A second index of inhibition in children over 5 years of age is contained in the reluctance to talk spontaneously to an unfamiliar examiner in a laboratory testing situation. The two most sensitive variables are latency to utter the first few spontaneous comments to the examiner (a comment is not a reply to an examiner's probe or question), and total number of spontaneous comments. This index of inhibition, which was gathered at both 5½ and 7½ years of age for Cohort 1, and at 5½ years of age for Cohort 2, was positively correlated with the earlier indexes of inhibition. When the index of inhibition derived from the peer play situation was averaged with the index of inhibition based on the testing context, the resulting standard score was correlated with each of the three earlier indexes of inhibition ($r = .67$, .54, .57 with the indexes at 21 months, 4 years, and 5½ years respectively; $p < .001$).

It is of interest that more inhibited children are later rather than first born (about two-thirds) and more uninhibited children are first born. Of the many possible interpretations, one is that later born status is more stressful for that small group of infants who are born with a biological disposition to become uncertain and aroused to unfamiliarity and challenge. An infant born with such a temperamental disposition might react with limbic arousal and withdrawal to the mild, but unexpected, intrusions of an older sibling who seizes a toy or teases the young infant.

As part of the assessment at 5½ years, the mothers were interviewed for factual information about the child. One part of that interview contained questions about the child's fears. The interviewer first let the mother describe the child's fears spontaneously. After the mother's spontaneous answers, the interviewer asked the mother to rate each of 10 fears on a 3-point scale, where a score of 1 indicated the fear was infrequent (no more than once in the last year), and a score of 3 indicated the fear was frequent (five or more times during the past year). The 10 fears were: large animals; being left alone in the house for a short time; fire; a large body of water such as a lake or ocean; elevators; machines; unfamiliar children; going to school for the first time; lightning or thunderstorms; and monsters on television or in movies. Inhibited children with a high and stable heart rate were more likely to have at least two fears (91% in contrast to 58%, 30%, and 70% of the other groups; chi square $=8.3$, 3 *df*, $p < .05$). Additionally, extreme fearfulness with unfamiliar children or fear of going to school (mother gave the child a rating of 3 for the items) was more common among the inhibited children with a high and stable heart rate than among the other three groups. Further, over half of these children were afraid of monsters in movies or on television and one-third had unusual fears or night terrors. One child was afraid of Santa Claus, another of a kidnapper coming to the home, and several were afraid of going alone to their rooms at night. Not one of the uninhibited children had any of these atypical fears; their fears were usually of large animals or the dark.

PHYSIOLOGICAL CHARACTERISTICS

We believe that the consistently inhibited children have lower thresholds of excitability in those limbic structures, especially the amygdala and hypothalamus, which serve the related psychological states social scientists call *uncertainty* or *anxiety*. As a result, the inhibited children are likely to show enhanced activity in the pituitary-adrenal axis, reticular activating system, and the sympathetic arm of the autonomic nervous system, as well as behavioral inhibition to unfamiliar or challenging events that cannot be assimilated. We first consider some physiological signs of sympathetic activity.

Heart Rate and Variability. We measured the child's heart rate and heart-rate variability to baseline and cognitive tasks on every assessment. Heart-rate variability was defined as the average standard deviation of the interbeat intervals across a series of episodes. Inhibited children had both higher heart rates (lower heart periods) and lower heart-rate variabilities at all ages, although at 7½ years the group differences were smaller than they were from 2 to 5½ years of age. However, differences in heart rate and heart-rate variability were preserved to a moderate degree across all the assessments. In Cohort 1 heart rate was preserved from 21 months to 7½ years ($r = .62$, $p < .01$), and in Cohort 2, from 31 months to 5½ years ($r = .59$, $p < .01$). Differences in heart-rate variability were also preserved to a significant degree across all assessments in both Cohorts ($r = .54$ from 21 months to 7½ years in Cohort 1; $r = .61$ from 31 months to 5½ years in Cohort 2). In addition, a sleeping heart rate obtained on Cohort 1 at 7½ years of age was significantly related to contemporary heart rate in the laboratory ($r = .49$, $p < .05$), as well as to the heart rate gathered in the laboratory at the three earlier ages ($r = .37$, .40, & .61 at 21 months, 4 years and 5½ years respectively, $p < .05$). The sleeping heart rate was not related to the aggregate index of inhibition at 7½ years, but was associated with the index of inhibition based on play with an unfamiliar child at 5½ years ($r = .35$, $p < .05$).

The children's heart rates tended to track their behavior over time. Among the inhibited children in Cohort 1, 11 of the 12 who remained inhibited across all assessments showed a consistently high or an increasing heart rate over the four assessments, in contrast to three of 10 inhibited children who became less inhibited over time. Among the uninhibited children, 5 of 7 who became slightly more inhibited showed high or rising heart rates over the assessments, in contrast to only 3 of 12 uninhibited children who remained uninhibited. A comparison of the consistently inhibited children and the consistently uninhibited children and the inhibited children who became less inhibited, on the other, yielded a significant chi square (6.2, $p < .05$).

Further, the consistently inhibited children had significantly higher heart rates than the consistently uninhibited children; these two behaviorally consistent groups had the highest and lowest heart rates respectively at every one of the assessments. For the less consistent groups, the inhibited children who became less inhibited showed a drop in heart rate between 5½ and 7½ years, whereas the uninhibited children who became inhibited showed a rise in heart rate over these two ages. As an uninhibited child becomes more shy, his or her heart rate rises; as an inhibited child becomes more outgoing, his or heart rate becomes lower.

Pupillary Dilation. Pupillary dilation is a second index of sympathetic activity, and the inhibited children in both the cohorts had significantly larger pupillary dilations to cognitive tasks than the uninhibited children. However, the pupil data were not as discriminating of the two groups as heart rate or heart-rate variability.

Voice. Projections from limbic structures to the skeletal muscles of the larynx and vocal cords are also at a higher level of activity in inhibited children.

Increased tension in these muscles is accompanied by a decrease in the variability of the pitch periods of vocal utterances (Stevens & Hirano, 1981). This increased tension can be due not only to discharge of the nucleus ambiguus but, indirectly, to sympathetic activity that constricts arterioles serving the muscles of the larynx. Because the vocal cords do not maintain a steady rate as they open and close, perturbations in the rate is a consequence of many factors, one of which is the tension in the laryngeal muscles. In her doctoral research, Coster (1986) reported that inhibited children in Cohort 1 at 5½ years had less variability of the pitch periods of single word utterances spoken under psychological stress than did uninhibited children.

Cortisol. Assessment of activity in the pituitary–adrenal axis required assays of unbound cortisol from saliva gathered at 5½ years of age in the laboratory as well as at home on three mornings before breakfast. The average cortisol level across the three home samples was significantly correlated with the original index of inhibition. However, it is of interest that when home cortisol levels on Cohort 1 were obtained 2 years later, at 7½ years, their discriminating power was less. Current stress, especially problems in school, was a better predictor of home cortisol levels than the original temperamental classification at the older age.

Although the inhibited children in the first cohort showed the peripheral physiological states to be expected from the hypothesis of lower thresholds of reactivity in the limbic system, only about one-third of the group showed signs of high activity in all of the target systems. Most of the correlations among the individual variables were low and nonsignificant. The statistical independence of these separate variables is a typical finding in the literature (see Nesse et al., 1985). We computed an aggregate index of responsivity across the separate indexes by computing a mean standard score for eight physiological variables quantified on Cohort 1 at 5½ years. The eight variables were: (a) cortisol level in the morning at home, (b) cortisol level in the laboratory, (c) heart rate during cognitive tasks, (d) heart-rate variability during cognitive tasks, (e) pupillary dilation during cognitive tasks, (f) variability of the pitch periods of vocal utterances, (g) standard deviation of all the fundamental frequency values and, (h) total norepinephrine activity based on a laboratory urine sample. A high standard score reflected greater limbic arousal. The correlations between the mean of the eight physiological variables and each of its component scores ranged from .36 to .56. The relation between this physiological aggregate and the index of behavioral inhibition at each age was highest with the original index of inhibition at 21 months ($r = .70$), but significant at the two later ages (.66, .58 with the indexes at 4 and 5½ years of age). It is of interest that the inhibited children who became less inhibited by age 5½ had lower physiological indexes than those who remained inhibited.

However, at 7½ years cortisol levels gathered at home did not differentiate the two groups as clearly. We believe that the cortisol levels gathered at 7½ years may reflect current environmental stress in addition to temperamental disposition. School represents a major stress for young children and about one-half of the formerly inhibited children with higher cortisol levels were experiencing serious psychological problems in school, even though they were not the most timid 7½ year olds. By contrast, none of the inhibited children with low cortisol values was having school problems, as reported by the mother, even though some were very shy. These facts suggest that contemporary sources of uncertainty that have not been defended against successfully are associated with high cortisol levels. It appears that, with school entrance, environmental factors independent of temperament can begin to influence the limbic structures and functions that we believe are the origins of changes in these psychophysiological variables. Thus, there are two reasons why the cortisol and the heart rate levels might be less differentiating of the two groups at older ages than they were earlier. As uninhibited children leave the home and encounter new stressors they can develop changes in limbic excitability and, as a result, show higher heart rates and higher cortisol levels. It is also possible that some children that have been consistently shy and timid for 6 years may have developed an automatized response profile that is more independent of the limbic state that supported it originally. If such children do not encounter new chronic sources of major uncertainty in their lives, limbic arousal (and, therefore, heart-rate and cortisol levels) may come to approximate levels found in the average child.

We also found some cognitive performances that may reflect limbic arousal. One sensitive psychological index of the state of uncertainty created by an adult examiner is deterioration in recall memory performance. At 5½ years of age inhibited children showed a larger loss in recognition memory accuracy than uninhibited children following a series of difficult cognitive tests. At 7½ years of age we implemented a test of recall memory. Each child listened to a 3-minute long taped voice narrate a story. At the completion of the story the child was given 18 chromatic pictures and asked to arrange the pictures to match the chronology of the story. After a series of intervening cognitive tests, a parallel version of the recall memory test was administered. A significantly larger proportion of inhibited (59%) than uninhibited (31%) children showed poorer performance on the second than on the initial recall memory test (chi square $= 3.1$, $p < .05$; the remaining children showed no change or an improvement in memory).

A second psychological procedure administered at 7½ years affirms the idea that uncertainty generated by stimulus events can impair cognitive performance in inhibited children. Each child was shown 32 pairs of chromatic pictures of people, animals, or objects and was told that for some pairs the two pictures were identical, whereas for others they differed in a subtle way. One half of the pictures were similar and one half different. The child had to decide if the pair of pictures was identical or different and to indicate the nature of the difference. One half of the pictures were neutral in content and the other half were emotional in content (a person bleeding; a person tied up with a rope). We assumed that the emotional content would generate greater uncertainty in the inhibited than in the uninhibited children. As predicted, more inhibited than uninhibited children made more errors on the emotional than on the neutral scenes (73% vs. 36%, chi square $=5.4$, $p < .05$), but there were no group differences in performance on the neutral scenes.

Iris Pigmentation and Behavioral Inhibition. We have also found that the children in both cohorts who remained behaviorally inhibited over the many assessments were more likely to have blue than brown eyes. In addition, the proportions with blue eyes rose if the children were both inhibited and had stable heart rates. In Cohort 1, 57% of the children who were inhibited and also had high and stable heart rates had blue eyes, whereas 36% of this group had brown eyes. In Cohort 2 the comparable proportions were 64% and 36%. By contrast, the consistently uninhibited children who had low and variable heart rates were most likely to have brown eyes. When the two cohorts were combined the resulting chi square was significant (7.3, $p < .01$). It is of interest that independent data from other samples support this association. In a longitudinal, but unpublished, study of a normative sample of children seen at 14, 20, and 32 months in our laboratory, Reznick found a significant association between consistently inhibited behavior and blue eyes. Finally, Rosenberg and Kagan (1987) found this association in cross-sectional samples of 269 children, from 133 kindergarten through third-grade classrooms, who had been nominated by their teachers to represent the extremes on the two behavioral dimensions. More children nominated to be extremely sky had blue eyes; more children nominated as extremely sociable had brown eyes (chi square $=7.7$, $p < .01$) .

There are several mechanisms that can serve as a foundation for explaining a relation between eye pigment and the temperamental qualities of inhibition and lack of inhibition to the unfamiliar. The first assumes a correlation between the amount of melanin in the eye and the amount of neuromelanin in the central nervous system and appeals to evidence indicating that neuromelanin has a modulating role in catecholaminergic transmission. High levels of neuromelanin should be associated with lower levels of central norepinephrine. As a result, limbic thresholds should be higher. A second class of explanation attributes a critical role to the pituitary peptide proopiomelanocortin (POMC), and its derivative, alphamelanocyte stimulating hormone (alpha MSH). Alpha MSH is a melanotrophic substance that may also function as a neuromodulator to raise thresholds of limbic activity as well as facilitate melanin dispersal in the iris. A final possible explanation, perhaps the most likely, assumes that the association between blue eyes and inhibition is the result of higher levels of central norepinephrine, which would lower thresholds of limbic arasol and sympathetic reactivity while simultaneously blocking the dispersal of melanin (see Rosenberg & Kagan, 1987, for details).

The Role of Norepinephrine. The temperamental qualities we have called *inhibition* and *lack of inhibition* to unfamiliar events seem moderately stable over time and have reasonable correlates with peripheral physiological responses, implying a lower threshold of activation in the amygdala and related parts of the limbic system. The correlations between behavior and the physiological signs hovered near 0.5, but varied a great deal. Therefore, we view the peripheral physiological signs—heart rate, heart-rate variability, cortisol, pupillary dilation—as imperfect indexes of the central state we are trying to understand and measure. The heightened physiological responsivity among inhibited children could be due to special structural characteristics in parts of the limbic system or in their projections, greater responsivity of the target organs, or differences in brain biochemistry that influence thresholds in the limbic system and, in turn, affect the probability of discharge of the stress circuits. Although each of these mechanisms is possible, current research favors the latter hypothesis.

One reasonable, albeit hypothetical, argument holds that the locus coeruleus, a brain stem structure that is the main source of central norepinephrine, produces more of this neurotransmitter in inhibited children. If this were true, the limbic system, especially the amygdala, would be at a higher level of excitability and prone to discharge to slight increases in uncertainty or challenge (Charney & Redmond, 1983). Kopin (1984) has suggested that genetic differences in the amount of norepinephrine secreted to anticipated stress among different animal strains may be analogous to differences in proneness to anxiety among humans. Charney, Heninger, and Breier (1984) believe that increases in central norepinephrine are causally related to attacks of panic anxiety in human patients.

Panic Patients. There may be a modest relation between temperamentally based inhibition in childhood and risk for agoraphobia, or for the more extreme diagnosis of panic disorder, in adulthood. Panic patients, who typically are women, report being extremely anxious as children and experiencing fear of leaving home and going to school because it required separation from the mother (Berg, 1976, Gittleman & Klein, 1984; Raskin, Peeke, Dickman & Pinsker, 1982). Additionally, panic patients have higher heart rates and lower finger temperature (Freedman, Ianni, Ettedqui, Pohl, & Rainey, 1984), and higher levels of epinephrine, norepinephrine, and cortisol (Nesse et al., 1985) than patients from other diagnostic categories. Some investigators have hypothesized that panic attacks might be due to increased central noradrenergic activity attributable to the action of the locus coeruleus. The increase in plasma MHPG levels when panic patients are in fear arousing situations is viewed as supportive of this idea (Ko et al, 1983). There is also support for the proposition that agoraphobia and panic are heritable, for about 25% of the relatives of panic patients (vs. 2% for controls) have a form of anxiety disorder (Harris, Noyes, Crowe, & Chaudry, 1983), and twin studies imply a genetic contribution to panic attacks, but not to generalized anxiety (Torgersen, 1983). These facts, together with the finding that imipramine has a therapeutic effect on panic but little or no benevolent effect on general anxiety disorder, imply a specific biological contribution to panic symptoms that might be similar to the mechanisms that mediate temperamentally based inhibited behavior in children.

Animal Models. Recent research with cats comes closer to specifying the role of the limbic system in inhibited behavior. Adamec and Stark–Adamec (1986) have found that domestic cats (Felis catus) display considerable variation in the tendency to be defensive to novelty and nonaggressive with rats. This variation in defensiveness emerges during the second postnatal month, and once the individual bias to be either defensive or aggressive has appeared it remains stable for many years. The defensive cats who do not attack rats are also inhibited when placed in an unfamiliar room, with a familiar human in an unfamiliar environment, or when they hear the tape recording of conspecific threat vocalizations. Further, the defensive cats show greater piloerection, larger pupillary dilation, and more trembling—all signs of sympathetic arousal—when exposed to unfamiliar incentives. Although specific experiences early in life (e.g., rearing with conspecifics who serve as models for killing rats, periodic food deprivation, and exposure to killed prey) facilitate adult aggressive behavior, even within a group of cats who have experienced these same facilitating conditions, there will be a group who will not attack rats (Adamec, Stark-Adamec, & Livingston, 1983).

Careful developmental observations have revealed that the average kitten first approaches prey at about 22 days, a few days before it will display withdrawal to the same incentive (about 27 days). However, the kittens who will become nonaggressive adults show a larger than normal increase in withdrawal behavior at 1 month, whereas the kittens who will become aggressive adults fail to show this exaggerated rise in withdrawal.

The appearance of withdrawal in the kitten at the end of the first month has a parallel in the appearance of similar behavior in wolf pups at the same age, fearfulness in monkeys at 2 months, and stranger anxiety in human infants at about 7 months of age. These remarkable concordances in the age when withdrawal and/or emotional distress to novelty emerge imply that particular forms of postnatal maturation of the brain are necessary before a state of uncertainty to novelty can mediate defensive behavior. It may not be a coincidence that the period from 1 to 2 months in the kitten corresponds to the time when the amygdala begins to modulate the hypothalamic substrate that may help to mediate defensive behavior (Kling & Coustan, 1964).

This corpus of facts led Adamec and his colleagues to perform a series of experiments suggesting that the responsiveness of the amygdala and hypothalamus is associated with defensive behavior. Defensive cats, compared with the aggressive animals, have a lower threshold of seizure susceptibility in the amygdala and greater propagation of seizure activity from the amygdala to the thalamus and hypothalamus. The more defensive the cat, the stronger the evoked neural response in areas to which the amygdala projects, especially the ventromedial nucleus of the hypothalamus. In addition, while orienting to a rat, defensive cats show more prolonged increases in neural activity in both amygdala and hypothalamus. Finally, repeatedly induced electrical evocation of after discharges in the perforant path of the ventrohippocampal system produced defensive behavior in ordinary nondefensive cats for periods as long as 30 to 60 days. This induced defensiveness appeared to be mediated by an increase in excitability of synaptic transmission between the amygdala and the hypothalamus (Adamec & Stark–Adamec, 1983; Adamec, Stark–Adamec, & Livingston, 1983).

Changes Between 5 and 7 Years. The hypothesis that changes in limbic excitability over time make a contribution to the preservation of inhibited or uninhibited behavior may be related to our observation that between 5½ and 7½ years of age there was a significant increase in the consistency of both inhibited and uninhibited behavior during the visits to the laboratory. Children who were still inhibited at 7½ years were much more consistent across all the testing contexts than they had beeen 2 years earlier. And it was these consistently inhibited children who showed the physiological signs described earlier. Many psychologists have reported more robust preservation of personality characteristics after age 6 than before (Kagan & Moss, 1962), inviting the speculation that biological changes occurring between 5 and 7 years of age mediate stabilization of the qualities of inhibition and lack of inhibition.

One of the processes that might contribute to the stabilization of inhibited behavior involves the idea of limbic kindling. A brief, daily burst of electrical stimulation to the amygdala of rats or cats leads to permanent sensitization of this structure. After 30 to 60 days of daily 1-second bursts of stimulation, animals begin to show spontaneous limbic convulsions, even though the electrical stimulation has ceased. If inhibited children are born with a more excitable amygdala, a frightening environmental event might function as a kindling stimulus. The anxiety-arousing events in daily life might include thunderstorms, marital quarrels, attacks from a sibling, or violent television shows. Such events, occurring three or four times a week over 5 to 6 years, could act as kindling stimuli for inhibited children and could make them susceptible to spontaneous attacks of anxiety. Several inhibited children at 7½ years did display unprovoked bouts of fear. On a particular day such a child would announce that he or she was reluctant to go to school or to go upstairs to sleep in the evening. Adult panic patients also report being behaviorally inhibited as children and a sudden panic attack in a department store could be regarded as analogous to a spontaneous limbic seizure in a kindled animal.

The Meaning of Inhibition. The evidence that we used as the referents for the predicates inhibited and uninhibited changed with age and, as a result, the meanings of the constructs changed. The primary behaviors defining inhibition at 21 months were clinging to the mother, crying, and retreat from unfamiliar incentives, responses that were rare at the later ages. The primary indexes at age 4 were a long latency to initiate contact with the unfamiliar peer and sitting or standing near the mother for long periods of time. At 5½ years of age, when we assessed the children in four very different contexts, only 3 of the 10 correlations among the five principle indexes were statistically significant, and even these significant correlations were modest (range of .30 to .45). An aggregate index of inhibition, representing the mean standard score across each of the five situational indexes, was positively correlated with each of its five component scores, but showed the highest relation to the child's reluctance to contact the novel objects in the unfamiliar room (r =.73) and the lowest correlation with behavior in the school setting (r =.37). The difference in magnitude of relation suggests that the processes mediating the initial reaction to a very novel situation may be different from the processes mediating social behavior in a more familiar context. The correlation between the two variables was only .22.

The possibility that the concept of *inhibition* may refer to two psychological qualities that are only moderately related is also supported by the heart rate data gathered during administration of the cognitive tests. The child's absolute heart rate in the laboratory was significantly associated with time proximal to the mother, reluctance to play with the unfamiliar peer during the first 10 minutes of the peer play session, and failure to play with all of the novel toys in the unfamiliar room. These behaviors seem to reflect an initial restraint in an unfamiliar situation. However, heart rate was not correlated with the child's reluctance to talk to the examiner over the 90-minute testing session or with social behavior with peers at school (r =.06, .21). The latter two variables seem to reflect lack of sociability in a more familiar context. Thus, the predicate inhibition appears to have two slightly different theoretical meanings at 5½ years.

The Role of Historical Information. The stability correlations for behavioral inhibition across the assessments ranged between 0.5 and 0.6. Thus, a proportion of children changed their ranks on the behavioral indexes, even though we had originally selected behaviorally extreme children at 21 or 31 months.

The group play data gathered at 7½ years, illustrated in Fig. 7.1, provide a

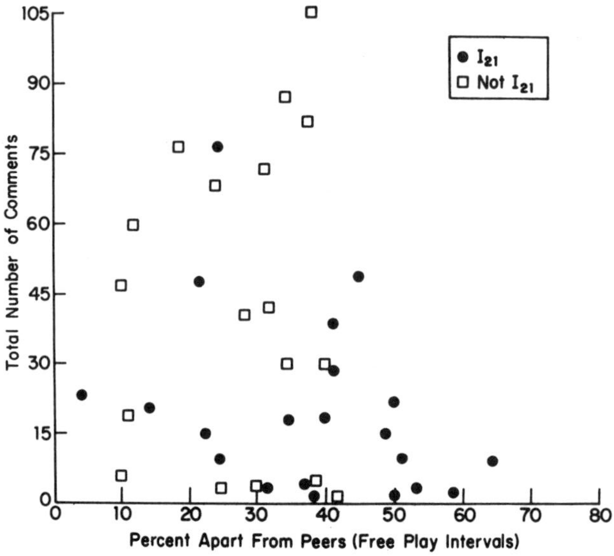

FIG. 7.1 Scatter plot of the total number of spontaneous comments made by each child and percent of time the child played apart from another child during the free-play intervals in the group play situation at 7½ years: Cohort 1.

result of theoretical interest. Of 21 children who had been classified as behaviorally inhibited at 21 months, the scores of 2 boys on the two major variables (total spontaneous comments and percent time apart from any other child during the free-play intervals) were similar to the mean scores of the uninhibited children. Of 18 children who had been classified as uninhibited at 21 months, 2 girls were as behaviorally inhibited as a typical inhibited child.

These results engage the perplexing problem of classification in the natural sciences. Evolutionary biology provides an analogy. The group called *pheneticists* argue that similarities in contemporary characteristics are the only important taxonomic criteria. However, *cladists* argue that similarities in phyletic origin should be the primary criteria. Mayr (1982), along with other biologists, has suggested that both evolutionary history as well as current similarities are to be used in classification. We suggest this rule is also useful in personality. As noted, two boys classified as inhibited at 21 months were, at 7½ years, not distinguishable from boys originally classified as uninhibited on two important variables. Should we ignore our knowledge of their early characteristics and classify them as uninhibited at 7½ years? We suggest a negative answer in this particular case, because neither boy was similar to the modal uninhibited child on other variables regarded as theoretically relevant to the two constructs. One boy showed a loss in reconstructive memory performance after the intervening cognitive stressors. The other boy had a high and stable heart rate. Both qualities are typical of inhibited, but not uninhibited, children. Indeed, no child classified originally as inhibited or uninhibited at 21 months had a profile on all of the theoretically significant variables gathered at 7½ years that was similar to any child in the complementary group (these variables are: heart rate, heart-rate variability, behavior with the peer, behavior with the examiner, and behavior on the cognitive tests). The longitudinal data from the second cohort of children selected at 30 months of age also support this conclusion. Two children who had been extremely inhibited at 30 months were uninhibited at 5½ years in both school and laboratory. Yet, both children continued to show a high and stable heart rate characteristic of inhibited children. By contrast, 2 children who had been classified as uninhibited originally became more inhibited, but continued to show the low and variable heart rates characteristic of uninhibited children.

Although investigators must remain receptive to the possibility that an individual can change his or her original psychological category, it is not clear what information will permit that judgment so that one can disregard knowledge of an individual's past. The pragmatist regards this question as metaphysical because one can never say with certainty that two objects belong to the same category. Someone may discover a feature, which had been disguised, that now distinguishes two groups that had appeared similar. Animal species that had been classified as closely related based on evidence from bone fragments are viewed currently as less closely related based on biochemical evidence.

However, many current investigations in personality and social psychology do not try in a minimal way to discover bases for differentiating among individuals who have similar values on one or two dependent variables. I suspect that if psychologists systematically gathered data on three variables that are crude indexes of a person's earlier experiences; namely, ordinal position, ethnicity, and education of the subject's parents (in addition, of course, to the sex of the subject), a sufficiently large proportion of the time they would discover at least two categories of individuals with different profiles of scores on the outcome variables. It is also likely that, having parsed their sample into subgroups, the results of the study would be interpreted more easily. For example, when the distribution of IQ scores from school-age children who had been born premature are compared with those of normal children, conclusions about the consequences of prematurity are very different for children growing up in middle-class versus lower class families. A second example comes from our research, for later born inhibited children with older siblings are more likely to remain inhibited over the preschool years than inhibited children who are first born or only children.

When a profile of qualities is considered ahistorically, the scientist is tempted to regard the summary predicate as reflecting a stable characteristic. When assessments of change are attempted or acknowledged one is less likely to conceive of the predicate as naming a stable essence. No popular construct in contemporary personality communicates accurately the changing profiles of behavior and heart rate displayed by the children in Cohort 1 across the period from 21 months to 7½ years. If the investigator focuses on one profile at one moment in time—a freeze frame—it is tempting to conceptualize inhibition as a fixed characteristic. The addition of historical information thaws the frozen moment and persuades one of the utility of categories that are more fluid.

The problem of inventing terms for transitional states has not been addressed in a serious way by psychologists who study personality development. Scientists in other domains frequently invent words to describe transitional states. A person recovering, but not yet recovered, from an illness is *in remission*; categories like *unbound cortisol* or *neutrino* refer to transition states. But it is less common to find category terms in personality that name classes of individuals who possessed all of the primary qualities of a category at one time, but only some of those qualities at a future time. One reason for the indifference to transition categories is the reluctance to gather historical data directly or obtain information that has indirect implications about the past.

The current data imply the need for at least four related constructs to capture the different psychological states associated with inhibition and lack of inhibition. One predicate refers to a biologically based predisposition, present at birth, that renders a child likely to develop one of the profiles, should the proper environmental experiences occur during the first year or two of life. The second term captures the meaning of inhibition or lack of inhibition as we have used it in this chapter; that is, the display of restraint, caution, and shy behavior, or their absence, in most unfamiliar contexts. A third descriptor is needed to describe the child who has changed some components of the above defining profile. The boy who became behaviorally uninhibited in the play contexts at 7½ years but retained a high and stable heart rate characteristic of inhibited children provides an example. The argument for the fourth predicate, which is more hypothetical, rests on the assumption that some children might lose completely their biological predisposition to be inhibited or uninhibited as a result of intervening experiences (some children who had been allergic to ragweed or milk for many years lose their allergic sensitivity later in life). I believe it is possible for some inhibited children to gain control of the processes that predispose them to be restrained and shy. No child in our study has met the criteria for this category, but it remains a real possibility.

SUMMARY

All infants born with an easily excited amygdala do not become inhibited children. The temperamental vulnerability requires chronic environmental stressors if the behavioral disposition is to be actualized. Some possible stressors include frequent hospitalizations, chronic parental quarreling, or serious economic privation that generates tension in the home. Most of our children did not experience these stressors. However, as we noted, a large number of inhibited children had older siblings. The presence of an older sibling who unexpectedly seizes a toy or yells at the younger child might provide the chronic stress necessary to actualize the infant's diathesis. An infant not born with these temperamental characteristics would not be as stressed by the same social experiences. Finally, it is necessary to differentiate between shy, introverted adolescents who are endogenously prone to uncertainty because they belong to our temperamentally inhibited group, and shy adolescents who acquired their behavior profile during the school years as a result of experience and who are not temperamentally prone to uncertainty. The likelihood of reversibility in behavior is greater for this second group. Use of selected physiological indexes, including heart rate, cortisol, pupillary dilation, and vocal tension might permit investigators to differentiate between these two classes of children.

ACKNOWLEDGMENTS

This research was supported in part by grants from the John D. and Catherine T. MacArthur Foundation and grant 40619 from the National Institute of Mental Health.

REFERENCES

Adamec, R. E., & Stark-Adamec, C. (1983). Partial kindling and emotional bias in the cat: Lasting effects of partial kindling of the ventral hippocampus. *Behavioral and Neurobiology, 38*, 223–239.

Adamec, R. E., & Stark-Adamec, C. (1986). Limbic hyperfunction, limbic epilepsy, and interictal behavior. In B. K. Doane & K. E. Livingston (Eds.), *The limbic system*, (pp. 120–145). New York: Raven.

Adamec, R. E., & Stark-Adamec, C., & Livingston, K. E. (1983). The expression of an early developmentally emergent defensive bias in the adult domestic cat in non–predatory situations. *Applied Animal Ethology, 10*, 89–108.

Berg, I. (1976). School phobia and the children of agoraphobic women. *British Journal of Psychiatry, 128*, 86–89.

Blizard, D. A. (1981). The Maudsley reactive and non-reactive strains. *Behavioral Genetics, 11*, 469–489.

Bronson, W. C. (1981). *Toddlers' behaviors with age mates*. Norwood, NJ: Ablex.

Charney, D. S., & Redmond, D. E. (1983). Neurobiological mechanisms in human anxiety. *Neuropharmacology, 22*, 1531–1536.

Charney, D. S., Heninger, G. R., & Breier, A. (1984). Noradrenergic function in panic anxiety. *Archives of General Psychaitry, 41*, 751–763.

Conley, J. J. (1985). Longitudinal stability of personality traits: A multi–trait multi–method multi–occasion analysis. *Journal of Personality and Social Psychology, 49*, 1266–1282.

Coolidge, J. C., Brodie, R. B., & Feeney, B. (1964). A ten year follow–up study of 66 school phobic children. *American Journal of Orthopsychiatry, 34*, 675–684.

Coster, W. (1986). *Aspects of voice and conversation in behaviorally inhibited and uninhibited children.* Unpublished doctoral dissertation, Harvard University, Cambridge, MA.

Cranach, B. V., Grote-Dahm, R., Huffner, U., Marte, F., Reisbeck, G., & Mitterstadt, M. (1978). Das Social Gehemmte Kind in Kindergarten, *Praxis der Kinderpsychologie Und Kinderpsychiatrie, 27,* 167–179.

Eaves, L., & Eysenck, H. (1975). The nature of extroversion: A genetical analysis. *Journal of Personality and Social Psychology, 32,* 102–112.

Freedman, R. R., Ianni, P., Ettedgui, E., Pohl, R., & Rainey, J. M. (1984). Psychophysiological factors in panic disorder. *Psychopathology, 17,* 66–73.

Garcia-Coll, C., Kagan, J., & Reznick, J. S. (1984). Behavioral inhibition in young children. *Child Development, 55,* 1005–1019.

Gittleman, R., & Klein, D. F. (1984). Relationship between separation anxiety and panic and agoraphobic disorders. *Psychopathology, 17,* 56–65.

Goldsmith, H. H., & Gottesman, I. I. (1981). Origins of variation in behavioral style: A longitudinal study of temperament in young twins. *Child Development, 52,* 91–103.

Gottesman, I. I. (1963). Heritability of personality, *Psychological Monographs,* whole no. 372, 1–26.

Harris, E. C., Noyes, R., Crowe, R. R., & Chaudry, D. R. (1983). Family studies of agoraphobia. *Archives of General Psychiatry, 40,* 1061–1066.

Jung, C. G. (1924). *Psychological types.* New York: Harcourt Brace.

Kagan, J., Kearsley, R., & Zelazo, P. (1978). *Infancy: Its place in human development.* Cambridge: Harvard University Press.

Kagan, J., & Moss, H. A. (1962). *Birth to maturity.* New York: Wiley.

Kagan, J., Reznick, J. S., Clarke, C., Snidman, N., & Garcia-Coll, C. (1984). Behavioral inhibition to the unfamiliar. *Child Development, 55,* 2212–2225.

Kagan, J., Reznick, J. S., & Snidman, N. (1987). The physiology and psychology of behavioral inhibition. *Child Development, 58,* 1459–1473.

Kling, A., & Coustan, D. (1964). Electrical stimulation of the amygdala and hypothalamus in the kitten. *Experimental Neurology, 10,* 81–89.

Ko, G. N., Elsworth, J. B., Roth, R. H., Rifkin, B. G., Leigh, A., & Redmond, D. E. (1983). Panic induced elevation of plasma MHPG levels in phobic anxious patients. *Archives of General Psychiatry, 40,* 425–430.

Kopin, J. J. (1984). Avenues of investigation for the role of catecholamines in anxiety. *Psychopathology, 17,* 83–97.

Loehlin, J. C. (1982). Are personality traits differentially heritable? *Behavior Genetics, 12,* 417–428.

Matheny, A. P. (1980). Bayley's infant behavior record: Behavioral components in twin analyses. *Developmental Psychology, 51,* 1157–1167.

Mayr, E. (1982). *The growth of biological thought.* Cambridge, MA: Harvard University Press.

Morris, D. P., Soroker, E., & Burruss, G. (1954). Follow-up studies of shy, withdrawn children I: Evaluation of later adjustment. *American Journal of Orthopsychiatry, 24,* 743–754.

Nesse, R. M., Curtis, G. C., Thyer, B. A., McCann, D. S., Huber-Smith, M., & Knopf, R. F. (1985). Endocrine and cardiovascular responses during phobic anxiety. *Psychosomatic Medicine, 47,* 320–332.

Plomin, R. (1986). *Development, genetics and psychology*. Hillsdale, NJ: Lawrence Erlbaum Associates.

Raskin, M., Peek, H. V. S., Dickman, W., & Pinsker, H. (1982). Panic and generalized anxiety disorders. *Archives of General Psychiatry, 39*, 687–689.

Reznick, J. S., Kagan, J., Snidman, N., Gersten, M., Baak, K., & Rosenberg, A. (1986). Inhibited and uninhibited behavior: A follow-up study, *Child Development, 51*, 660–680.

Rosenberg, A., & Kagan, J. (1987). Iris pigmentation and behavioral inhibition. *Developmental Psychobiology, 20*, 377–392.

Schneirla, T. C. (1959). An evolutionary and developmental theory of biphasic processes underlying approach and withdrawal. In M. R. Jones (Ed.), *Nebraska Symposium on Motivation*. Lincoln: University of Nebraska Press.

Schneirla, T. C. (1965). Aspects of stimulation and organization in approach-withdrawal processes underlying vertebrate development. In D. S. Lehrman, R. A. Hinde, & E. Shaw (Eds.), *Advances in the study of behavior* (Vol. 1, New York: Academic Press, pp. 1–74).

Scott, J. P., & Fuller, J. L. (1974). *Dog behavior: The genetic basis*. Chicago: University of Chicago Press.

Snidman, N. (1984). *Behavioral restraint and the central nervous system*. Unpublished doctoral dissertation, University of California, Los Angeles, CA.

Stevens, K. N., & Hirano, M. (Eds.). (1981). *Vocal fold physiology*. Tokyo: University of Tokyo Press.

Stevenson-Hinde, J., Stillwell-Barnes, R., & Zunz, M. (1980). Subjective assessment of rhesus monkeys over four successive years. *Primates, 21*, 66–82.

Suomi, S. J. (1984). The development of affect in rhesus monkeys. In N. A. Fox & R. J. Davidson (Eds.), *The psychology of affective development* (pp. 119–159). Hillsdale, NJ: Lawrence Erlbaum Associates.

Thomas, A., Chess, S. (1977). *Temperament and development*. New York: Brunner Mazel.

Torgersen, S. (1983). Genetic factors in anxiety disorders. *Archives General Psychiatry. 40*, 1085–1089.

8

The Development of Coping Responses During Adolescence: *Endocrine and Behavioral Aspects*

Anne C. Petersen
Elizabeth J. Susman
John L. Beard
The Pennsylvania State University

The consideration of how individuals cope with uncertainty requires examination of the development of coping responses. Whereas some degree of uncertainty has always been a part of life, there is likely to be age-related variability in the nature and extent of uncertainty experienced by the individual. Furthermore, individual variability is likely to exist in the responses to uncertain situations. An important question, then, is, "What develops?" We could, at one extreme, propose that coping responses are entirely learned. Alternatively, we could propose that all that changes developmentally is the nature of uncertainty that is experienced by the individual, with the coping responses determined by inherited characteristics. Most likely, however, the "truth" lies somewhere between these extremes. The capacity to feel aroused, responsivity to arousal, and behavioral coping repertoires are likely to change through childhood and adolescence. Biological changes in arousability, other developmental changes in cognitive and affective capacity, learning that gives meaning to arousal, and age-related changes in the nature of uncertainty experienced are all likely to affect the responses of an individual to some uncertain circumstances or situation.

We begin with a conceptual frame for biopsychosocial development (see Fig. 8.1) that considers the development of interacting systems, between individuals and important social contexts as well as between biological and behavioral processes within the individual. Such macrodevelopmental processes may be differentiated from microprocesses involving change in biological–behavioral interactions over brief time periods at a single developmental age or phase. Such microprocesses—for example, between adrenal hormones and behavior—may be uniform at all ages or, alternatively, may themselves develop or change with

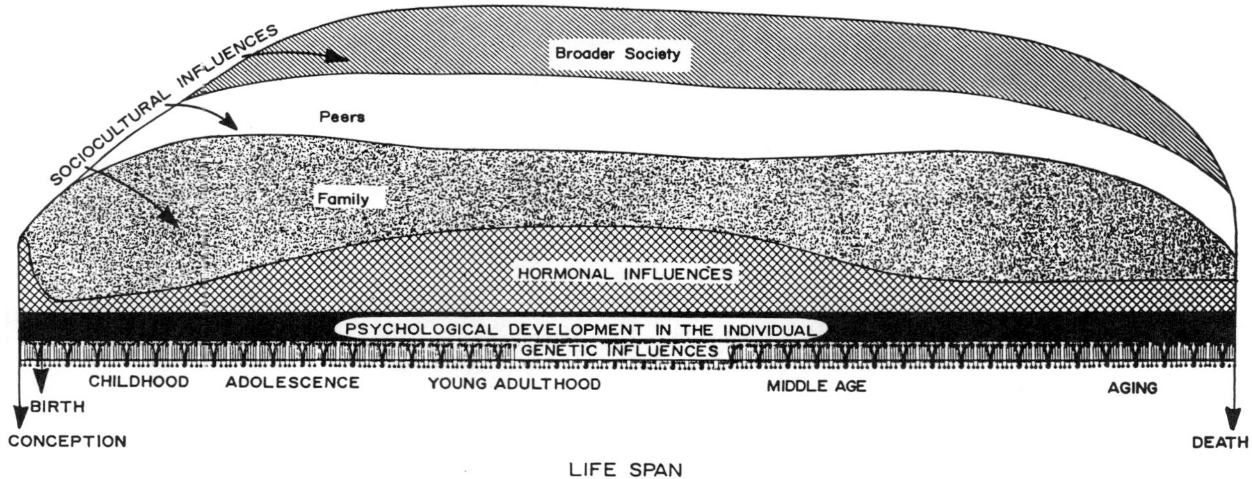

FIG. 8.1 Some factors hypothetically influencing psychological development over the life span (from Petersen, 1980).

increasing maturation of the individual. We also assume that, in general, biological and behavioral factors are typically two aspects of the same process rather than one aspect (e.g., biology) inevitably causing the other aspect (e.g., behavior). With specific process sequences, of course, one aspect *may* cause the other.

Much of the research related to the questions we address in this chapter has typically been labeled *stress research* (e.g., Petersen & Spiga, 1982). Consideration of developmental processes reveals the deficiencies or gaps in this body of work. For example, given that uncertainty is ubiquitous in life, is it inevitably stressful? The answer is clearly "no"; some uncertainty generates excitement and anticipation. For this reason, we prefer to consider the "challenge" of a situation rather than stress. A positive response to a challenge—for example, stimulation—may lead to positive change and growth. Challenges may, however, be overwhelming and experienced as stressful, leading to negative developmental patterns. Responses to challenge may be influenced by the individual's prior state (e.g., nutritional well-being); by the extent, duration, and nature of the challenge; and by the individual's physiological and cognitive/affective systems, with some predictable gender differences in the nature of coping responses. The usual model in stress research is to assume that the processes among these factors are uniform across age. But there is substantial evidence that all elements vary with developmental age or phase. We exemplify this point with evidence at adolescence.

COPING WITH ADOLESCENCE

Research on adolescent development has burgeoned in the last decade (cf. Petersen, 1988), with substantial information now available on the characteristics of development during the second decade of life. Now that at least some basic descriptive information now exists, a second generation of more process-oriented research has begun (e.g., Susman et al., 1987, in press).

What the evidence thus far makes clear is that adolescence is a challenging period of life. Adolescents experience change in every aspect of individual development and in every important social context (e.g., Petersen & Spiga, 1982). Some of these changes are listed in Table 8.1. Experiencing so much change within a brief period, such as early adolescence, may exacerbate typical responses. We describe some of the evidence for the role of a challenging period of life, early adolescence, in the development of coping responses.

Some research suggests that the extent of challenge in early adolescence produces divergence in developmental patterns of psychological functioning at this age (e.g., Petersen, Ebata, & Graber, 1987). Previously, it was thought that pubertal hormones caused normative adolescent turmoil (e.g., Kestenberg, 1968). Several lines of research have now demonstrated that this hypothesis was incorrect, at least in its simplistic form. First, not all adolescents manifest significant turmoil (e.g., Bandura, 1964; Offer & Offer, 1975). Therefore, a

TABLE 8.1
Developmental Stresses of Adolescence

Individual	
Puberty	Adult appearance and size
	Reproductive capacity
	Timing (especially if deviant)
	Internal endocrine changes
	Asynchrony (among body parts, among adolescents)
Cognitive	Capacity for abstract thought
Psychological	Development of identity
Social Context	
Peer groups	Conformity
	Pressure to try new experiences
School	Changing school structure and format
Parents	Parental responses to adult size of adolescent
	Sexual stimulation
	Implications for parent's aging
	Impending separation
Society	Hopes and expectations for youth
	Occupational choices and opportunities

universal change such as puberty is unlikely to be the cause of specific psychological difficulties. Second, except for one study (Rutter, 1980), most research finds no link between becoming pubertal and manifesting turmoil or psychological problems (e.g., Crockett & Petersen, 1987). Specific pubertal changes, however, may play a causal role with some individuals, a point we pursue later. Third, difficulties in adolescence are not transient but rather typically foretell diagnosable problems in adolescence or young adulthood (Rutter, Graham, Chadwick, & Yule, 1976; Wiener & Del Guadio, 1976). Therefore, the onset of puberty is unlikely to cause inevitable psychological problems. However, puberty involves major and significant changes in the lives of young adolescents.

Nevertheless, the prediction of significant psychological problems should improve in early adolescence, but not only because of puberty. Rather, the number and nature of all changes experienced at this age together with the individual's capacity to cope with challenge predicts the direction of subsequent development. This hypothesis is portrayed in schematic form in Fig. 8.2. We find, for example, that girls are more likely to experience difficult challenges and to cope less effectively with challenge compared to boys (Petersen & Ebata, 1987).

DEVELOPMENTAL CHANGE IN ADOLESCENCE

During early adolescence, significant changes occur in every aspect of individual development and in every important social context. All of this change creates a context of uncertainty for young adolescents and those who interact with them.

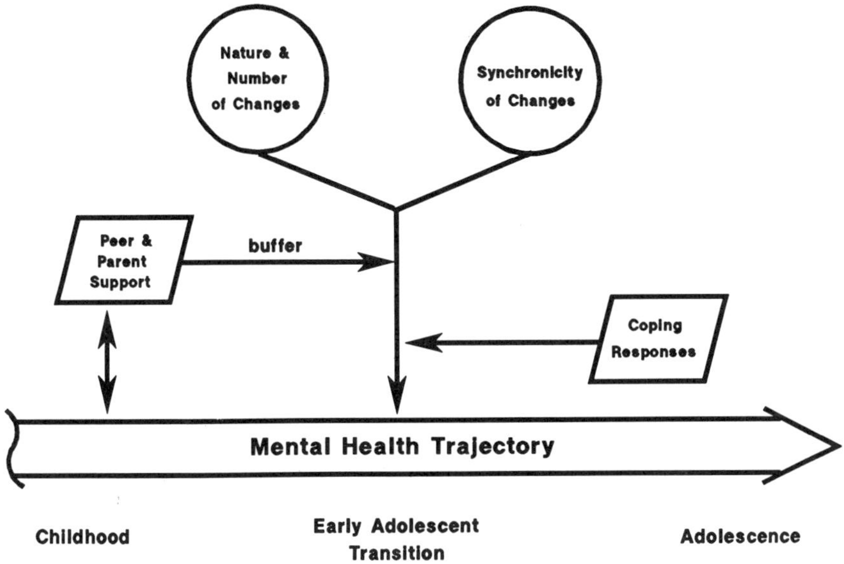

FIG. 8.2. A model of developmental transitions.

Two changes are probably most important, at least in the United States: the biological changes of puberty, and the change from an elementary school format to a secondary school format. The first change is within the individual and the second change is within a major social context. The several other changes may be considered derivative of or secondary to the pubertal and school changes. For example, the peer group is affected by both school and pubertal changes, with the school change altering the peers available to form a peer group, and puberty affecting heterosocial interactions and peer comparisons. The family and society are similarly affected by biological and social confirmation of the child's maturation. Cognitive development, particularly the capacity to think abstractly that begins to emerge in early adolescence, may be independent of puberty and school changes but the research evidence is insufficient here.

Puberty

The biological changes of puberty are striking in extent and occur fairly rapidly, changing the child into a person of mature appearance within 4 years on average (Tanner, 1974). (See Fig. 8.3 for the sequence of changes in boys and girls.) The internal endocrine changes begin a few years prior to the appearance of external manifestations. For girls, most of the observable changes take place between 10 and 15 years of age, whereas for boys the span is typically 11 to 16 years (Marshall & Tanner, 1969, 1970). Besides attaining adult size and appearance,

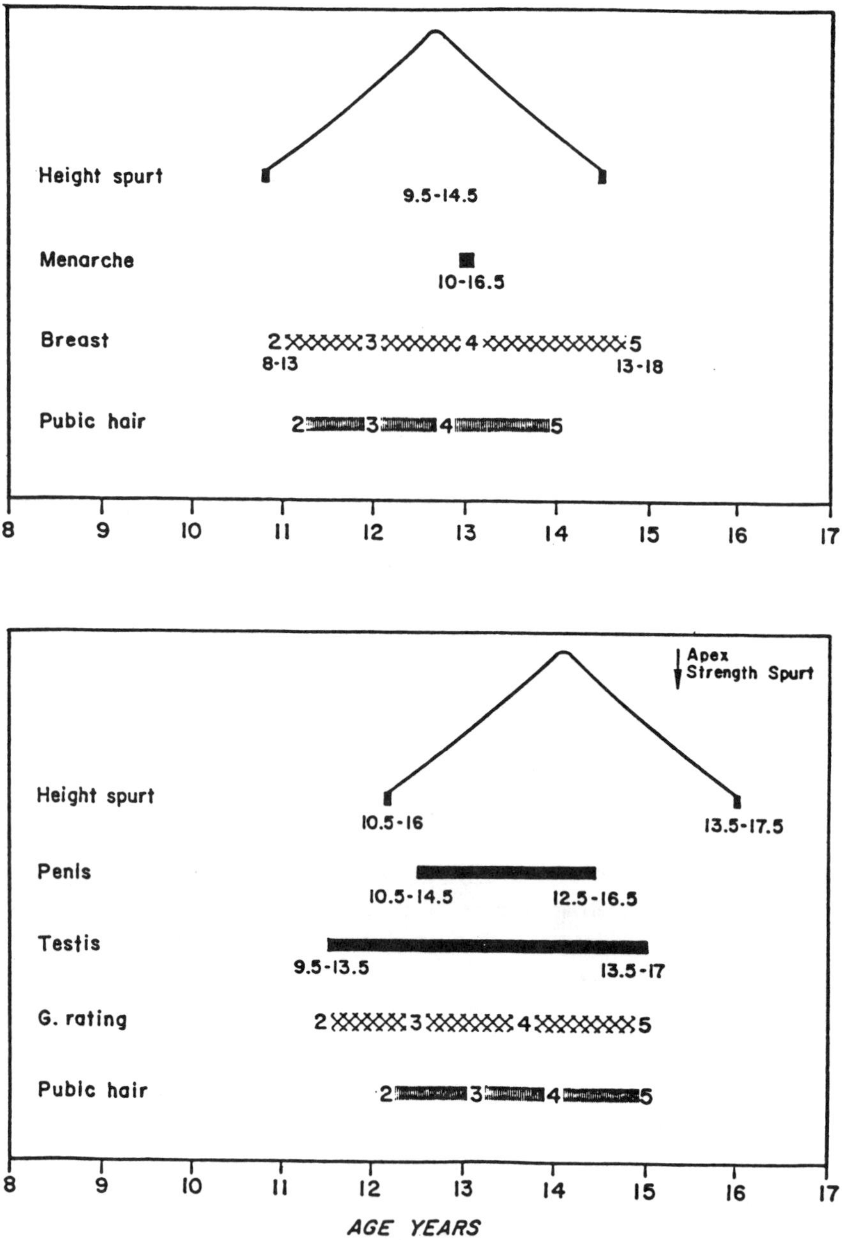

FIG. 8.3. Schematic sequence of somatic change at puberty for an average girl (upper) and boy (lower). The range of ages within which each change may begin and end is given by the numbers placed directly below the start and end, respectively, of each one (from Tanner, 1974).

youngsters develop reproductive capacity during puberty; this involves the development of the menstrual cycle in girls and the development of viable sperm in boys.

Pubertal change and its timing are highly variable between individuals, adding to the feelings of uncertainty of this age. Even within the individual, the sequence and timing of change in specific characteristics may be highly variable (Eichorn, 1974). For example, in one girl all the changes may occur fairly synchronously, whereas in another they may change gradually and sequentially. In one boy, the testes may develop first, whereas in another pubic hair might be the first manifestation. All of these variations lead young adolescents to feel somewhat anxious about what they will experience, with what outcome, and whether their changes are normal.

Apart from the normal individual differences in variations in the timing and duration of puberty, there are some predictable sources of influence. A major factor of relevance here is the effect of inadequate nutritional intake, particularly combined with intense physiological demands, on the growth process. Dancers, for example, who restrict their diets and exercise intensely several hours per day, have delayed menarche and longer limbs when compared to sisters and mothers (Brooks-Gunn & Warren, 1987). Similar results have been seen in undernourished individuals of both sexes: Puberty begins later and is prolonged.

The rapid physical growth of puberty increases demands for adequate nutrients to support this maturation (Tanner, 1974). The acute or chronic lack of adequate nutrition constitutes another "stressor" that is unlikely to have a positive outcome. Even if the individual has the benefit of adequate nutrition at some later point in development, and therefore "catches up" in physical growth and reproductive capacity, the consequences of inadequate nutrition at the time of greatest growth are likely to extend to cognitive and affective capacities, affecting the young person's ability to experience normative developmental changes and growth in school and relationships. These experiences are more difficult than physical growth to address at a later point in life. Research examining these issues would be quite valuable.

School Change

School change is usually more uniform for youngsters within a local community but still may have variable effects on individuals. From school to school, the nature of changes involved in the transition from elementary to secondary format is also variable. More constant features of this school transition include the movement from a small, neighborhood school with a single teacher and a single group of classmates to a larger, geographically more distant school involving a different teacher and set of classmates for each subject area or course. Simmons and Blyth (1987) have characterized the secondary school environment as more anonymous for the individual, a factor that is likely to increase uncertainty.

These two changes—puberty and school changes—are identified as having major importance because of their direct impact on the developing adolescent and because of their effects on other changes. For example, puberty results in an adult-sized individual with mature reproductive capacity, both factors with major social significance. An example of school changes affecting other contexts is with the peer group. A larger school involves a larger peer group. This context change is associated with changes in friendship.

Early adolescence, then, may be characterized as a developmental period involving more uncertainty for the individual. In addition to these normative developmental changes in early adolescence, nonnormative changes occur at this age with predictable frequencies. For example, death or illness of family members, parental divorce, and economic changes in the family all occur for young adolescents. Some family changes occur with increased frequency for young adolescents relative to children, especially parental divorce, parental death, and mothers working outside the home. The increased number of changes has a direct effect on the individual's well being (e.g., Simmons &Blythe, 1987; Simmons, Burgeson, Carlton-Ford & Blyth, in press). Furthermore, the experience of increased change can affect all youngsters in the cohort, whether or not they personally experience lots of change.

COPING RESPONSES IN ADOLESCENCE

All of the changes just described create a great deal of uncertainty in early adolescence. Although some of the changes are completed in a few years, beginning the adolescent decade with so much change creates an atmosphere of uncertainty for the entire period. How, then, do adolescents cope with uncertainty? Although little research exists to inform this question, we will address the conceptual issues in terms of endocrine responsivity, brain development, behavioral development, and their interactions.

Basic Neuroendocrine Processes

It is not yet known whether the gonadal hormone system has different effects on behavior at the outset of puberty than in the mature organism but there is some reason to believe that the effects are different. The issue is whether a uniform amount of hormone has different effects in organisms at different developmental statuses. Brooks-Gunn and Warren (1987) reported recently that estrogen levels were related to depressed mood in girls right around the time of menarche, suggesting that the brain may be differentially responsive to a particular level of hormone early in the pubertal process compared to brain responsivity later in development. Because of the recency of endocrine studies in adolescence, hormone-behavior studies have not been feasible until recently; therefore, much more research is yet needed.

Until recently, the adrenal cortical hormone system was thought to be fairly independent of the gonadal hormone system. Although these systems manifest different developmental patterns, with cortisol levels, for example, fairly constant across developmental periods, it is now known that these two endocrine systems are interrelated, with reciprocal effects.

The brain probably continues growing and developing until around puberty, with the fastest growth earlier in life (Graber & Petersen, in press). Cell regeneration, of course, is a lifelong process but new cell growth beyond that needed for replacement appears to take place in the brain only in the earlier part of the life cycle. There are few studies of neural growth among adolescents in particular so evidence for the nature of growth at this time is fairly speculative. Most scholars believe that neural organization is fairly stable by the end of puberty, based on evidence that damage is severe thereafter. Because of effects of experience on the brain, however, the observed pattern of growth could reflect experience (e.g., schooling) as well as underlying neural maturation.

Developmental Change in Behavioral Responses

Coping responses in early adolescence may be altered by two related processes. First, behavior may be altered by direct hormone effects on central nervous system functioning that, in turn, may affect behavior. The brain is a target tissue for some puberty-related hormones (e.g., estrogen). Second, behavior may be altered indirectly by physical maturation changes. Changes in height, weight, and body proportions are a stimulus to adolescents themselves and to others of the adolescent's more mature status. This new status means that adolescents are exposed to increasing demands for more independent and responsible behavior. In brief, at puberty, changes in hormone levels may alter the brain biochemical milieu such that behavior is altered. Changes in hormone levels also are responsible for changes in physical maturation that, in turn, may affect coping and adjustment.

At a folk wisdom level, hormones long have been implicated in the behavior changes that occur during adolescence. At an empirical level, hormones as influences on adolescent behavior were not the focus of study until recently. (See Susman, Nottelmann, Inoff-Germain, Dorn, & Chrousos, 1987, for a review of hormones and behavior in adolescence.) When the role of hormones was considered, pituitary–gonadal axis hormones and their manifestations, physical maturation and reproductive function, were the presumed causal influences on behavior. Specifically, gonadal steroids were linked to changes in aggression at puberty (Olweus, Mattsson, Schalling, & Low, 1980).

The hypotheses linking the increase in androgens at puberty and the increase in aggression during human adolescence grew out of past studies showing consistent associations between androgen levels and aggressive behavior in male animals and somewhat less consistent links in female animals (Bouissou, 1983; Eleftherious & Sprott, 1975). In human adolescents, published reports from at least two studies link levels of puberty-related hormones and aggressive behavior. In the first study, Olweus and colleagues (Olweus et al., 1980) reported that in male adolescents higher levels of testosterone were related to higher levels of aggressive behavior. Testosterone also appeared to have an indirect causal influence on provoked aggression with low frustration tolerance as a mediating variable (Olweus, 1986). A high level of testosterone was interpreted as making a boy impatient and irritable which, in turn, may lead to unprovoked and destructive aggression.

In a second, more recent study, higher testosterone levels, as well as androgens of adrenal origin, were hypothesized to be related to mother-reported levels of aggressive attributes in male and female adolescents (Susman et al., 1987). Emotional dispositions (irritability, anxiety, and sadness) were hypothesized to be involved in the pathways between hormone levels and aggression. The general pattern of findings was that a profile of lower gonadal steroid levels and higher androstenedione levels was related to acting out and rebellious behavior. Specifically, lower estradiol, testosterone to estradiol ratio, testosterone–estradiol binding globulin, and dehydroepiandrosterone sulphate were associated with more acting out behavior problems. Higher levels of androstenedione, an androgen of adrenal origin, was also associated with more acting out behavior problems. Feeling nervous or anxious was the emotional disposition related to acting out behavior problems. The findings relating hormones, emotional dispositions and aggressive attributes were reported only for boys.

In another aspect of the same study, Nottelmann and colleagues (Nottelmann, Susman, Inoff-Germain, Cutler, Loriaux, & Chrousos, 1987) reported that the profile of lower levels of gonadal steroids and higher levels of adrenal androgens also was associated with indices of psychosocial adjustment, as well as to aggressive behavior. The pattern of findings between indices of psychosocial adjustment problems and indices of physical maturation—chronological age, pubertal status, and serum hormone levels—was examined. For boys, in particular, adjustment problems were associated with a hormone profile that is typical of later maturation: relatively low gonadal steroid levels, or lower pubertal stage, frequently in conjunction with higher chronological age. Higher androstenedione levels also were related to more adjustment problems. In brief, adjustment problems were higher in males with lower pubertal stage for chronological age and lower gonadal steroid levels for chronological age. For girls, the findings were fewer and less consistent. Adjustment problems for girls were associated with higher levels of gonadotropins, lower levels of dehydroepiandrosterone sulphate, and higher levels of androstenedione, sometimes in combination with lower pubertal stage.

The profile of lower gonadal steroid levels and higher levels of androstenedione together with aggressive behavior, negative emotions, and adjustment problems identified in young adolescents is consistent with a similar profile reported in studies of animals and human adults encountering endogenous and exogenous stressors. The profile of lower levels of hormones of gonadal origin and higher levels of hormones of adrenal origin is illustrative of the interaction between the endocrinology of reproduction with the endocrinology of the stress response (see Collu, Gibb, & Ducharme, 1984). The implications of the interaction between these two systems, the hypothalamic-pituitary-gonadal axis (HPG) and the hypothalamic-pituitary-adrenal axis (HPA), for human development are discussed in detail in this volume (see Susman, Nottelmann, Dorn, Gold, & Chrousos, this volume). Briefly, with regard to adolescence, coping with the other challenges of adolescence (e.g., changes in peer and family relationships) may result in chronic adrenal activation as reflected in higher levels of androstenedione. Other hormones associated with adrenal cortical activation, increased levels of corticotropin releasing factor, adrenocorticotropin hormone, and cortisol, may suppress the gonadal axis, in turn, leading to delayed physical maturation and reproductive function (Nottelmann, Inoff-Germain, Susman, & Chrousos, in press). An alternative interpretation is that later maturers may experience chronic levels of stress because of their delayed physical maturation, as reflected in lower levels of gonadal steroids. Immature appearance relative to that of same-age peers, and accompanying emotional sequelae, may constitute a stressor culminating in higher levels of adrenal cortical activation.

The interpretation of the pattern of findings described above is highly speculative because of the cross-sectional nature of the design. The unknown causal direction of the hormone-behavior processes involved in the findings cited above is representative of the many unanswered questions related to the causal direction of neuroendocrine changes of adolescence, environmental challenges of adolescence (e.g., changes in peer and family relationships), and the development of coping responses in adolescents. As we have suggested earlier, undoubtedly the causal influence of hormones on behavior changes or behavior on hormone changes are part of ongoing developmental processes rather than bidirectional causal influences unique to adolescence. What is unique about adolescence is that the puberty-related hormone changes that occur in early adolescence are much more rapid than the changes in hormone levels that occur in other periods of the lifespan. For instance, testosterone levels in males increase approximately 18-fold across the five stages of pubertal development (Nottelmann, Susman, Dorn, Inoff-Germain, Loriaux, Cutler, &

Chrousos et al., 1987), a period of development spanning approximately 5 years. Longitudinal studies of adolescents across the years while they are experiencing rapid puberty-related hormone changes provide the ideal, but yet to be utilized, design for testing hypotheses regarding the causal links between the neuroendocrine changes of puberty and behavioral development.

Environmental Challenges and Coping During Adolescence

Although it is assumed that the hormone changes of puberty and their manifestations, physical growth, and reproductive maturation, are inherently stressful, this assumption is far from being empirically verified. The same is true for the environmentally imposed social and emotional challenges and uncertainties of young adolescents. In general, we know neither what constitutes challenge or uncertainty for adolescents nor their behavioral and biological reactivity to specific challenges. Greater specificity is needed in defining: (a) situations and contexts that are inherently challenging to most adolescents, (b) individual differences in biological and behavioral reactivity to these challenges, and (c) implications of individual differences in reactivity to specific challenges for other aspects of social and emotional development (e.g., implications for the development of emotional or behavior problems).

The development of sophisticated models for studying reactivity to challenges and the development of coping in adolescents now seems feasible because of recent advances in the study of neuroendocrine and behavioral reactivity to stressors in animals (Levine, Wiener, Coe, Bayart, & Hayashi, 1987; Suomi, 1987), human infants (Gunnar, Isensee, & Fust, 1987; Tennes & Carter, 1973; Tennes, Downey, & Vernadakis, 1977), and young children (Kagan, Resnick, & Snidman, 1987; Tennes & Kreye, 1985). In contrast to past research, the recent focus has been on explaining the conditions under which neuroendocrine and emotional and behavioral factors are associated and dissociated, and the implications of these covariations for development. Earlier research used a simplistic model for integrating states of emotional arousal and neuroendocrine reactivity. Specifically, the most common approach was to correlate indices of arousal, primarily negative emotions, to indices of adrenal cortical activation, primarily cortisol levels. The recent studies of primates and humans also have been based on theories of child development as a way of conceptualizing individual differences in biological and behavioral reactivity to environmental challenges. For instance, the effects of mother-infant separation has been used as a paradigm for examining microanalytic processes involved in emotional arousal and adrenal cortical and adrenal medullary activation (Levine et al., 1987; Schanberg & Field, 1987). For instance, in rhesus macaques and squirrel monkeys, Levine and colleagues (1987) studied behavioral and hormonal sequelae of brief periods of mother-infant separation. Conditions under which there were both associations and dissociations between reactivity of the pituitary–adrenal system and vocalizations, considered an index of distress in primates, were identified.

Similarly, in a differentiated approach to arousal and endocrine activity in human infants, Gunnar and colleagues (1987) examined differences in the biomedical status of newborns as a moderating influence on adrenal cortical activity. Extremely healthy and normal newborns were compared with slight perinatal problem newborns on adrenal cortical activity and the Brazelton Neonatal Behavioral Assessment Scale with Kansas supplement (NBAS-K; Brazelton, 1973; Horowitz, Sullivan, & Linn, 1973). There were no associations between cortisol levels and NBAS–K for the extremely healthy and normal newborns. However, there were associations between peak of excitement, rapidity of buildup, irritability, tremulousness, and the summary score in the slight perinatal problem group. There were no mean level differences in cortisol levels or NBAS–K dimensions between the two biomedical status groups. Because of the different pattern of within-group cortisol and behavior associations, and the lack of group differences, the findings were interpreted as indicating that activity of the adrenal cortex is not apparently linked to a specific dimension of neonatal behavior. The behavior of the neonates may have been moderated by their biomedical state.

These studies elegantly demonstrated that a sophisticated and differentiated approach to the biological and psychological reactivity to stressors is essential before conclusions are warranted regarding emotional arousal and endocrine activity. If a similar, conceptually rich approach were applied to examining adrenal cortical and behavioral reactivity to environmental challenges in adolescents, consideration of the adolescent's biological traits and states hypothesized to regulate many behavioral states would be especially important to consider. Specifically, the biological states of early, middle, and late puberty are characterized by very different levels of hormones of gonadal and adrenal origin, as well as height, weight, and other morphological characteristics. The activational influences of hormones on central nervous functioning and hence, behavior, may be quite different for the different stages of puberty. In fact, evidence exists suggesting that progression through puberty indeed may alter metabolic processes in such a way as to alter many other physiological processes, such as those involved in drug metabolism (Hein, 1987). These same physiological processes also may be involved in alterations in reactivity to environmental challenges. In brief, a differentiated approach to the possibility of developmental differences in reactivity to environmental challenges may help to clarify the assumed but elusive connection between progression through puberty and the onset of mood alterations and variability and affective disorders in adolescents.

The separation–attachment situations used successfully in examining reactivity to challenges in infants and young children may be an especially appropriate context for examining biological and behavioral reactivity to the challenges of adolescents. Adolescence is the developmental period in which separation from family in order to gain independence and autonomy, and the development of new attachment relationships are major developmental tasks. In addition, it is the developmental period in which separation from friends may be especially emotionally arousing. In these separation–attachment situations, self-reports of emotional arousal and indices of adrenal cortical (cortisol), as well as adrenal medullary indices (cathecholamines or their metabolites), obtained concurrently, may produce findings that lead to a more sophisticated understanding of the reaction of adolescents to separation, an assumed environmental challenge for all age groups.

We offer one caveat when using models developed with animals or human infants and young children for conceptualizing similar phenomena with adolescents. The associations between the neuroendocrine and emotional indices of arousal may be altered by age-related developmental processes. Namely, adolescents learn ways of coping that are consistent with their chronological age (e.g., big boys don't cry). However, the degree of adrenal activity may not be associated with behavioral styles of coping. This line of thinking is inconsistent with earlier assumptions that adrenal cortical activity provides a window for observing degree of emotional arousal. When emotional arousal was found not to be consistently related to adrenal cortical arousal, the validity of cortisol level as a psychobiological index of stress came under question (see Gunnar, Marvinney, & Isensee in this volume). As demonstrated by Levine and colleagues (1987), one should not expect that adrenal corticol reactivity, as reflected in cortisol levels, and degree of emotional arousal necessarily should be consistently associated across behaviors and contexts. This speculation with regard to adolescents has received some support. Susman and colleagues (Susman, Dorn, Nottelmann, Inoff-Germain, & Chrousos, in preparation) reported that in response to the challenge of three phlebotomy procedures, over a 1-year period, young adolescents showed a significant decrease in distress behavior during the procedure. Cortisol levels did not decrease across the same period. These findings suggest that the phlebotomy procedure continued to be emotionally arousing, as reflected in cortisol levels. However, the adolescents appeared to have learned to cope with the situation by decreasing potentially embarrassing external displays of distress behavior, a coping strategy which is consistent with the developmental expectation that adolescents will exhibit mature and responsible behavior.

In conclusion, a common feature of the findings for both animals and humans cited above is the wide degree of individual variability in reactivity to environmental challenges. For adolescents, these individual differences may be even greater because of their accumulated experience in learning strategies for coping with environmental challenges, either as a consequence of inherited characteristics or learned coping strategies, may be one factor contributing to the increase in turmoil and behavior problems in some adolescents but not in others.

ADDITIONAL CHALLENGE IN ADOLESCENCE: THE EXAMPLE OF IRON DEFICIENCY

One of the examples whereby environmental "stressors" interact with developmental "stressors" may be that of the iron deficient adolescent. There are indications in the animal and human literature that iron deficiency affects neurotransmitter metabolism, adrenal–pituitary function, and behavior.

National health and nutrition surveys in both Canada (Seone, Roberge, & Page, 1985) and the United States (HANES II Survey, 1985) have revealed the existence of a new "at-risk" group for tissue iron deficiency and anemia. Adolescent boys, ages 11–14, were as much at risk for clinical iron deficiency as were women of reproductive age; around 11%, as defined by very low levels of serum ferritin. This biochemical indicator of iron status represents a measure of iron stores of the body. The absence of storage iron is associated most frequently with anemia, although it is now clear that other organ systems in the body that require iron for normal function are affected, in some cases, more severely than the red cell (Beard & Finch, 1985).

The causes of iron deficiency in adolescence are unclear, but in males it is suspected that the very high growth rates that occur at the peak growth spurt may require boys to increase essential body iron by over 50% in 12 months. It is probably the combination of limited dietary intake prior to, during, and perhaps after this spurt that depletes storage iron and begins limiting physiological function. The most clearly documented functional alterations in tissue iron deficiency are decreased physical work capacity, poor immune function, and altered thermoregulation (Dallman, 1986). The human literature also contains numerous reports of alterations in behavior and cognition in infancy, childhood, and during adolescence (Pollitt, 1986).

A common thread of observations of effects of iron deficiency on cognition appears to be related to attentional deficits. There are consistent and significantly decreased abilities of iron deficient children and adolescents to score well on learning achievement and task-oriented tests that measure concentration and attention (Pollitt, Loibel, & Greenfield, 1983). A recent study of adolescent pregnant girls showed a significant improvement in scores on the Digit Symbol test and on attention measures after a short period (8 weeks) of iron supplementation (Groner, Holtzman, Charney, & Mellits, 1986). These observations have been repeated in other cultural settings, such as rural Indonesia (Soementri, Pollitt, & Kim, 1985), Egypt (Scrimshaw, 1984), and Guatemala (Lozoff & Brittenham, 1986). In most cases, oral iron therapy (over a period of 2 to 3 months) resulted in a normalization of many of the cognitive measures (Matching Familiar Figures test and Raven Progressive Matrices tests). We would expect that measures of achievement may take longer to correct given the prolonged period during which nutritional deprivation could affect learning capacity. In the Groner study, cultural factors were not considered significant given the relatively short time of the dose and response. It is likely, however, that the improved performance on tests and tasks result from the removal of inhibitory influences of iron deficiency. Nearly all of these human studies suffer from measuring complex outcome variables and lack of specificity of measurement. It is the consistency of observation of abnormalities during iron depletion, however, that is convincing.

The biologic causality of these cognitive changes may relate to the essential role of iron in the metabolism of central nervous system (CNS) neurotransmitters. Iron is an essential cofactor in both the tryptophan and tyrosine hydroxylase enzyme systems and thus key to the synthesis of serotonin and the dopamine, epinephrine, and norepinephrine systems. Indeed, recent studies in rats show alterations in plasma norepinephrine levels that precede the detection of anemia during progressive iron depletion (Groeneveld, Smeets, Kabra, & Dallman, 1986). Although brain iron content is fairly well protected relative to other organs during depletion, very significant changes in CNS serotonin and dopamine content and metabolism are known to occur. Elevations in urinary norepinephrine, representing primarily peripheral sympathetic nervous system release and metabolism, are observed in iron deficient humans (Oski, Honig, Helu, & Howanitz, 1983). These elevated catechols returned to normal levels with iron treatment and, within the same time frame as, the normalization of certain cognitive tests. The fact that peripheral metabolism of neurotransmitters is altered, as shown by elevated plasma and urine norepinephrine in humans and tissue turnover in rats (Beard & Tobin, 1987), suggests the possibility that certain autonomic nervous system tasks like locomotion, metabolic rate, and temperature regulation are altered in iron deficiency. Thus, it is possible that not all of the alterations in cognition have their basis in central neural dysfunction, some part may be based on actual reception of stimuli from the environment, and the capacity to mount an appropriate skeletal muscle or metabolic response to that situation. It is clear that physical exercise capacity is limited in iron deficiency (Dallman, 1986), though we have often attributed this to a limitation in skeletal muscle oxidative capacity. Spontaneous activity in rats is diminished and contact time increased in infants are perhaps indications of this decreased capacity (Lozoff & Brittenham, 1986). It now seems reasonable to ask if the neural control of those processes might also be limiting as well. Indeed, the lack of ability of the iron deficient adolescent to perform well physically may limit self-esteem and socialization in a pathway somewhat distinct from a direct route suggested by the altered attentional capacities mentioned previously.

A second possible mechanism whereby iron deficiency mediates this poor cognitive performance is by representing a major biologic stressor (nonspecific to iron) that threatens the integrity of the cognitive machinery. Certainly, the early studies in Mexico of protein energy malnutrition demonstrate that nutritional stress itself causes a decrease in responsiveness to the environment, apparent apathy, and poor performance on cognitive tasks. It is not outside the realm of possibility that poor test performance and perceptual disturbances are related to a generalized nutritional deprivation and socioeconomic deprivation in addition to the direct effects of iron deficiency.

The third possibility represents a generalized stress-response reflex from the adrenal that may be exhibited by down regulation of the hypothalamic-pituitary-gonadal axis, down regulation of the adrenal cortex, and up regulation of the adrenal medulla. Substantive data to support any of the three of these possibilities are lacking, although the elevated urinary norepinephrine data from both rat and human studies argue for a specificity of response; that is, epinephrine levels are similar under control and experimental stress situations, whereas norepinephrine levels are elevated. Investigations are currently underway in both humans and rats to examine ACTH and cortisol responses to an exercise stressor.

A poor socioeconomic setting is positively correlated with iron deficiency in the United States. Limited nutrient intakes are commonly observed in adolescents in this situation. A long-term marginal intake and a short-term acute deficit prior to and during the adolescent growth spurt can potentially set up the likelihood of a tissue deficient adolescent. They may or may not have other environmental factors that limit cognitive development though it is highly probable that some difficulties in cognition and the development of certain skills will be limited by iron deficiency.

The high growth demands of adolescence thus sets up a scenario whereby iron deficiency can alter the individual's capacity to respond to stimuli by affecting the most basic of physical properties, neurotransmission. As an "environmental stressor" of both short- and long-term duration, iron deficiency may also reasonably affect the development of normal coping strategies in these growing individuals. It would be pure speculation to limit these comments to the adolescent since our interactive behavior with our environment could be altered by iron deficiency throughout the life span. Investigations are currently being planned to examine the relationship of iron nutriture to neurohormone metabolism, adrenal and gonadal hormones, and behavioral measures in an attempt to establish the significance of these potential interactions.

In summary, iron deficiency appears to dramatically alter activity and affective behavior (Lozoff & Brittenham, 1986), in addition to certain cognitive processes. The increased likelihood of iron deficiency during the adolescent growth spurt may have significant long-term functional consequences in a number of key areas of adolescent development.

SUMMARY

In this chapter, we have argued that the period of life called early adolescence is inherently challenging and becomes stressful for many young people. The amount of change experienced by most youngsters at this age exceeds their capacity to cope, stimulating some to develop more effective coping styles. Others, unfortunately, are likely to develop ineffective coping styles that may become lifelong patterns.

Several kinds of factors influence the amount of challenge experienced. Some youngsters reach early adolescence already weakened by prior experience, such as nutritional insufficiency. Those without family or social support or diminished in individual strengths (e.g., basic intelligence, good temperament) are likely to experience more difficulties (Ebata, 1987; Petersen & Ebata, 1987). Prior school failure is a major predictor of difficulties in early adolescence especially among boys (Ebata & Petersen, 1987). These results are consistent with previous research on stress and coping (e.g., Garmezy & Rutter, 1983).

The early adolescent experience itself varies significantly among individuals. Although an increased amount of change is experienced by all young adolescents, particularly because of the universal experience of puberty, and the likelihood of a major change of schools in the United States, some youngsters experience even more change than others. The sheer number of changes experienced is predictive of difficulties (Simmons et al., in press, 1987). In addition, too many simultaneous, rather than sequential changes can be stressful (Coleman, 1980; Petersen & Ebata, 1987). Finally, the nature of the changes is important. Some changes (e.g., parental death or divorce) have predictably more impact than others (e.g., parental job change).

The individual's response to challenge in early adolescence may be the most important developmental phenomenon to be examined. Given similar amounts and kinds of changes, why do some youngsters show negative effects while others may have neutral or even positive outcomes? Again, many factors must be considered. Prior learning about how to cope as well as learning acquired during early adolescence are surely important. As we have described, the physiological response system is important as well. There may be individual differences in arousability and resilience of the hypothalamic–adrenocortical system in the face of stress. Some may be able to respond calmly, or at least constructively to challenge, and use the potentially stressful experience to develop effective coping styles. Others may become overwhelmed, cognitively, physiologically, or both, and cope inadequately.

The example of iron deficiency, more likely to occur during early adolescence, provides a particularly interesting instance of a factor creating physiological, psychological, and cognitive stress on the individual. Serious alterations to the developmental pattern are likely to result.

If early adolescence represents a major developmental challenge for the development of effective coping, it is especially important to understand the influences on stress and coping responses. Research paradigms involving unusual stress, such as the study of iron deficiency, may be especially useful for identifying important factors, and ways to improve effective coping. In addition, the examination of those who do well in the face of excessive challenge, as well as those who fail to cope even under mild challenge should illuminate understanding of these processes.

REFERENCES

Bandura, W. (1964). The stormy decade: Fact or fiction? *Psychology in Schools, 1*, 224–231.

Beard, J. L., & Finch, C. A. (1985). Iron deficiency. In K. Weiner & F. Clyesdale (Eds.), *Iron fortification of foods* (pp. 3–16). New York: Academic Press.

Beard, J. L., & Tobin, B. (1987). Feed efficiency and norepinephrine turnover in iron deficiency. *Procdeeding Society for Experimental Biology and Medicine*, 337–344.

Bouissou, M. F. (1983). Androgens, aggressive behavior and social relationships in higher mammals. *Hormone Research, 18*, 43–61.

Brazelton, T. B. (1973). *Neonatal behavioral assessment scale* (Clinics in Developmental Assessment, No. 50). Philadelphia: Lippincott.

Brooks-Gunn, J., & Warren, M. (1987). *Biological contributions to affective expression.* Paper presented at the biennial meeting of the Society for Research in Child Development, Baltimore, MD.

Coleman, J. C. (1980). Friendships and the peer group in adolescence. In J. Adelson (Ed.), *Handbook of adolescent psychology* (pp. 408–431). New York: Wiley.

Collu, R., Gibb, W., & Ducharme, J. R. (1984). Effects of stress on gonadal function. *Journal of Endocrinological Investigations, 7*, 529–537.

Crockett, L. J., & Petersen, A. C. (1987). Pubertal status and psychosocial development: Findings from the early adolescence study. In R. M. Lerner & T. T. Foch (Eds.), *Biological–psychosocial interactions in early adolescence: A life-span perspective* (pp. 173–188). Hillsdale, NJ: Lawrence Erlbaum Associates.

Dallman, P. (1986). Biochemical basis of iron deficiency. *Annual Review of Nutrition, 6*, 13–34.

Ebata, A. T. (1987). *A longitudinal study of psychological distress during early adolescence.* Unpublished doctoral dissertation, The Pennsylvania State University, University Park, PA.

Ebata, A. T., & Petersen, A. C. (1987). *Patterns of adjustment during early adolescence: Gender differences in depression and achievement.* Manuscript submitted for publication.

Eichorn, D. H. (1974)., Asynchronizations in adolescent development. In S. E. Dragestin & G. H. Elder, Jr. (Eds.), *Adolescence in the life cycle.* New York: Halsted.

Eleftherious, B. E., & Sprott, R. L. (1975). *Hormonal correlates of behavior Vol. 1. A lifespan view.* New York: Plenum.

Garmezy, N., & Rutter, M. (Eds.). (1983). *Stress, coping, and development in children.* New York: McGraw Hill.

Graber, J. A., & Petersen, A. C. (in press). Cognitive changes at adolescence: Biological perspectives. In K. Gibson & A. C. Petersen (Eds.), *Brain maturation and behavior development: Biosocial dimensions.* Hawthorne, NY: Aldine de Gruyter.

Groeneveld, D., Smeets, H. G. W., Kabra, P. M., & Dallman, P. (1985). Urinary catecholamines in iron deficient rats at rest and following surgical stress. *American*

Journal of Clinical Nutrition, 42, 263–269.

Groner, J. A., Holtzman, N. A., Charney, E., & Mellits, E. D. (1986). A randomized trial of oral iron on tests of short term memory and attention span of young pregnant women. *Journal of Adolescent Health Care, 7*, 44–48.

Gunnar, M. R., Isensee, J., & Fust, L. S. (1987). Adrenocortical activity and the Brazelton neonatal assessment scale: Moderating effects of the newborn's biomedical status. *Child Development, 58*, 1448–1458.

Hanes II. (1985). *Health and nutrition evaluation survey report, 1976–1980.* Washington, DC: National Center for Health Statistics.

Hein, K. (1987). The interface of chronic illness and hormonal regulation of puberty. *Journal of Child and Adolescent Health, 8*, 530–540.

Horowitz, F. D., Sullivan, J. W., & Linn, R. (1973). Stability and instability in the newborn infant. The quest for elusive threads. In A. J. Sameroff (Ed.), Organization and stability of newborn behavior: A commentary on Brazelton neonatal behavior assessment scale. *Monographs of the Society for Research in Child Development, 43*, (5–6, Serial No. 177).

Kagan, J., Resnick, A., & Snidman, N. (1987). The physiology and psychology of behavioral inhibition in children. *Child Development, 58*, 1459–1473.

Kestenberg, J. (1968). Phase of adolescence with suggestions for correlation of psychic and hormonal organizations. Part III. Puberty, growth, differentiation, and consolidation. *Journal of the American Academy of Child Psychiatry*, 6, 577–614.

Levine, S., Wiener, S. G., Coe, C. L., Bayart, F. E. S., & Hayashi, K. T. (1987). Primate vocalization: A psychobiological approach. *Child Development, 58*, 1408–1419.

Lozoff, B., & Brittenham, G. M. (1986). Behavioral aspects of iron deficiency. *Program in Hematology, 14*, 23–53.

Marshall, W. A., & Tanner, J. M. (1969). Variations in the pattern of pubertal changes in boys. *Archives of Disease in Childhood, 44*, 291–303.

Marshall, W. A., & Tanner, J. M. (1970). Variations in the pattern of pubertal changes in boys. *Archives of Disease in Childhood, 45*, 13–23.

Nottelmann, E. D., Inoff-Germain, G., Susman, E. J., & Chrousos, G. P. (in press). Hormones and behavior at puberty. In J. Bancroft (Ed.), *Adolescence and puberty.* London: Oxford University Press.

Nottelmann, E. D., Susman, E. J., Dorn, L. D., Inoff-Germain, G., Loriaux, D. L., Cutler, G. B., Jr., & Chrousos, G. P. (1987). Developmental processes in early adolescence: Relations among chronological age, pubertal stage, height, weight, and serum levels of gonadtropins, sex steroids, and adrenal androgens. *Journal of Adolescent Health Care, 8*, 35–48.

Nottelmann, E. D., Susman, E. J., Inoff–Germain, G. Cutler, G. G., Jr., Loriaux, D. L., Chrousos, G. P. (1987). Developmental processes in early adolescence: Relations between adolescent adjustment problems and chronological age, pubertal stage and puberty-related serum hormone levels. *Journal of Pediatrics, 110*, 473–480.

Offer, D., & Offer, J. (1975). *From teenage to young manhood: A psychological study.* New York: Basic Books.

Olweus, D. (1986). Aggressions and hormones: Behavioral relationships with testosterone and adrenaline. In D. Olweus, J. Block, M. Radke-Yarrow (Eds.), *Developmental of antisocial and prosocial behavior: Research, theories, and issues* (pp. 51–72). Orlando, FL: Academic Press.

Olweus, D., Mattsson, A., Schalling, D., & Low, H. (1980). Testosterone, aggression, physical, and personality dimensions in normal adolescent males. *Psychosomatic Medicine, 42*, 253–269.

Oski, F. A., Honig, A. S., Helu, B., & Howanitz, P. (1983). Effect of iron therapy on behavioral performance in nonanemic, iron deficient infants. *Pediatrics, 71*, 877–880.

Petersen, A. C. (1980). Biopsychosocial processes in the development of sex-related differences. In J. Parsons (Ed.), *The psychobiology of sex-differences and sex roles* (pp. 31–55). New York: Hemisphere.

Petersen, A. C. (1988). Adolescent development. *Annual Review of Psychology, 39*, 583–607.

Petersen, A. C., & Ebata, A. T. (1987). Developmental transitions and adolescent problem behavior: Implications for prevention and intervention. In K. Hurrelmann, F. X. Kaufmann, & F. Losel (Eds.), *Social intervention: Potential and constraints* (pp. 167–184). Berlin and New York: Walter de Gruyter.

Petersen, A. C., Ebata, A. T., & Graber, J. (1987, April). *Responses to developmental and family changes in early adolescence.* Paper presented at the annual meeting of the American Educational Research Association, Washington, DC.

Petersen, A. C., & Spiga, R. (1982). Adolescence and stress. In L. Goldberger & S. Breznitz (Eds.), *Handbook of stress: Theoretical and clinical aspects* (pp. 515–528). New York: The Free Press.

Pollitt, E. (1986). Nutrition and intellectual performance. *Clinical Nutrition, 5*, 219–225.

Pollitt, E., Loibel, R. L., & Greenfield, D. B. (1983). Iron deficiency and cognitive test performance in preschool children. *Nutrition and Behavior, 1*, 137–146.

Rutter, M. (1980). *Changing youth in a changing society: Patterns of adolescent development and disorder.* Cambridge, MA: Harvard University Press.

Rutter, M., Graham, P., Chadwick, O., & Yule, W. (1976). Adolescent turmoil: Fact or fiction? *Journal of Child Psychology and Psychiatry, 17*, 35–36.

Schanberg, S. M., & Field, T. M. (1987). Sensory deprivation stress and supplemental stimulation in the rat pup and preterm human neonate. *Child Development, 58*, 1431–1447.

Scrimshaw, N. S. (1984). Functional consequences of iron deficiency in human populations. *Journal of Nutrition Science and Vitamins, 30*, 47–63.

Seone, N. A., Roberge, A. G., & Page, M. (1985). Selected indices of iron status in adolescents. *Journal Canadian Dietetic Association, 46*, 298–303.

Simmons, R., & Blyth, D. (1987). *Moving into adolescence: The impact of pubertal change and school context.* New York: Aldine.

Simmons, R., Burgeson, R., Carlton-Ford, S. L., & Blyth, D. (in press). Reaction to the cumulation of change in early adolescence. *Child Development.*

Soemantri, A., Pollitt, E., & Kim, I. (1985). Iron deficiency anemia and educational achievement. *American Journal of Clinical Nutrition, 42*, 1221–1228.

Suomi, S. J. (1987). Genetic and maternal contributions to individual differences in rhesus monkey biobehavioral development. In N. Krasnagor (Ed.), *Psychobiological aspects of behavioral development* (pp. 397–420). New York: Academic Press.

Susman, E. J., Dorn, L. D., Nottelmann, E. D., Inoff-Germain, B. E., & Chrousos, G. P. (in preparation). *Cortisol and behavioral reactivity in young adolescents.*

Susman, E. J., Inoff-Germain, G., Nottelmann, E. D., Loriaux, D. L., Cutler, G. B., &

Chrousos, G. P. (1987). Hormones, emotional dispositions, and aggressive attributes in young adolescents. *Child Development*, *58*, 1114–1134.

Susman, E. J., Nottelmann, E. D., Dorn, L. D., Inoff-Germain, G., Chrousos, P. (in press). Physiological and behavioral aspects of stress in adolescence. In G. P. Chrousos, D. L. Loriaux, & P. W. Gold (Eds.), *Physical and emotional stress: Biochemical mechanism and clinical implications*. New York: Plenum.

Susman, E. J., Nottelmann, E. D., Inoff-Germain, G., Dorn, L. D., & Chrousos, G. P. (1987). Hormonal influences on aspects pf psychological development during adolescence. *Journal of Adolescent Health Care*, *8*, 492–504.

Tanner, J. M. (1974). Sequence and tempo in the somatic changes in puberty. In M. M. Grumbach, G. D. Grave, & F. E. Mayer (Eds.), *Control of the onset of puberty* (pp. 448–470). New York: Wiley.

Tennes, K., & Carter, D. (1973). Plasma cortisol levels and behavioral states in early infancy. *Psychosomatic Medicine*, *35*, 121–128.

Tennes, K., Downey, K., & Vernadakis, A. (1977). Urinary cortisol excretion rates and anxiety in normal one-year-old infants. *Psychosomatic Medicine*, *39*, 178–187.

Tennes, K., & Kreye, M. (1985). Children's andrenocortical responses to classroom activities in elementary school. *Psychosomatic Medicine*, *47*, 451–460.

Weiner, I. B., & Del Guadio, J. M. R. (1976). Psychopathology in adolescence: An epidemiological study. *Archives of General Psychiatry*, *33*, 187–193.

9

Fundamental Systems of Emotion in the Mammalian Brain

Jeffrey A. Gray
Institute of Psychiatry, England

It is not my intention in this chapter to address directly developmental issues; I have neither clinical experience nor research data to render plausible such an intervention in a field not my own. Rather, I wish to present an outline sketch of what is known about those neuropsychological systems that, in the adult mammal (plausibly including humans), control emotional behavior. For I suppose that the work of developmental psychologists is likely to be aided by an understanding of the final product towards which the subjects they study are tending, and I also suppose that many of the abnormalities of behavior and development that concern the pediatric psychiatrist are emotional in nature.

BASIC ASSUMPTIONS

The sketch I present is underpinned by a number of basic assumptions.

The first is that emotions consist in specific states of the CNS, an abbreviation which stands simultaneously for the conceptual nervous system (Hebb, 1955), that is, the system deduced from purely behavioral analysis of the relations between stimulus input and response output, and the real central nervous system located inside the skull.

The second assumption is that emotions differ from other such central states in that they are elicited by reinforcing stimuli or events. In this context, the term *reinforcing stimuli* (and its congeners, *reinforcement*, *reinforcer*, etc.) has the standard definition common in learning theory (e.g., Gray, 1975), that is: Stimuli that, when made contingent upon a behavioral response, alter the subsequent probability of emission of that response, whether by increasing this probability (in which case the stimulus is a positive reinforcer or reward) or by decreasing it (making the stimulus a negative reinforcer or punishment). But note that this definition of a reinforcer refers to its response-*contingent* effects on behavior; in contrast, the definition of emotions offered here refers to the *eliciting* effects of reinforcing stimuli, that is, the changes they cause in central state and consequent behavior when a subject is exposed to them.

The third assumption is that specific emotional states differ from each other in the subsets of reinforcing events that elicit them and in the behavior to which each subset gives rise (Gray, 1972). In order to explicate this assumption we need first to consider the ways in which reinforcing events can be classified. An aid to such attempts at classification is presented in Fig. 9.1 (Gray, 1975). This shows that one may, contingent upon a response, either present, terminate, or omit (an otherwise expected) reinforcing stimulus, and that consequent upon such an experimental arrangement, one may observe either an increase or decrease in the probability of emission of the response concerned (if no change in response probability is observed, that means the putative reinforcer is not a reinforcer after all). As also shown in Fig. 9.1, it is an empirical generalization with a large

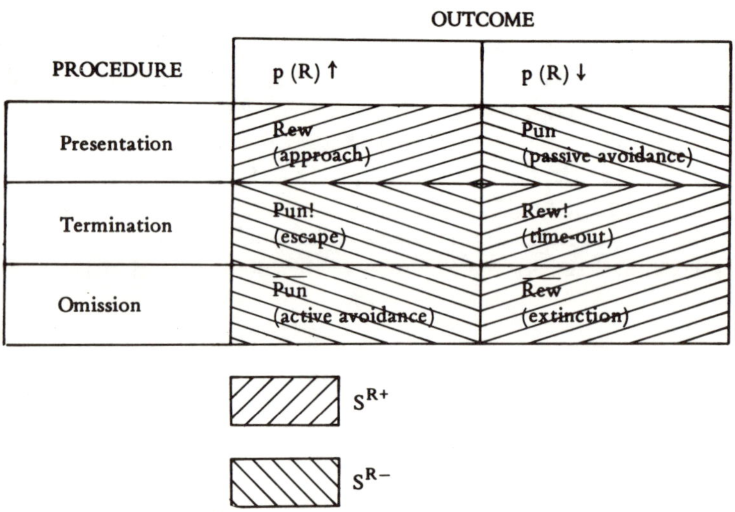

FIG. 9.1. A classification of reinforcing events. The abbreviation and symbols are as defined by the intersection of row (procedure) and column (outcome). *p(R)*↑:outcome is an increase in the probability of the response on which the reinforcing event is made contingent. *p(R)*↓:outcome is a decrease in the probability of this response. Crosshatching indicates those procedures–plus–outcomes which define a stimulus as an S^{R+} or an S^{R-}, respectively. Bracketed phrases refer to typical learning situations in which the various reinforcing procedures are employed. Rew: reward; Pun. Punishment; !. termination; —: omission.

measure of support that stimuli which increase response probability when presented contingently upon a response also decrease response probability when terminated or omitted response-contingently; similarly that stimuli which, when presented response–contingently decrease response probability also, when terminated or omitted, increase it. This is the basis for classifying stimuli as positive or negative reinforcers respectively. Thus, Fig. 9.1 offers three different ways of classifying reinforcing events, according to their mode of experimental arrangement (presentation, termination, or omission), to the observed change in response probability (increase or decrease), and to the use of a positive, or appetitive, reinforcer (reward) or negative, or aversive, reinforcer (punishment).

But the complications do not cease there. For Fig. 9.1 illustrates only the use of primary or unconditioned reinforcers, that is, stimuli that possess reinforcing properties for a given species without special learning (e.g., food, water, copulation). But, in addition, much of behavior is guided by secondary or conditioned reinforcers, that is, stimuli which initially have no reinforcing properties but which acquire them as a result of Pavlovian conditioning with a primary reinforcer serving as unconditioned stimulus. Such secondary reinforcers may be used in all the ways shown in Fig. 9.1 and, in general, they produce the same reinforcing effects as the primary reinforcers with which they have been associated by conditioning (Gray, 1975). However, as we see later, the emotional states they elicit differ in important respects from those elicited by primary reinforcers. Thus, in classifying reinforcing stimuli, we must also bear in mind the distinction between primary and secondary reinforcers.

A fourth assumption is that each emotional state that can be distinguished in terms of the type of behavioral analysis adumbrated in the previous two paragraphs will turn out to depend upon its own separable subsystem in the brain (Gray, in press); and, furthermore, that these "emotion systems" will be anatomically located largely in the limbic system rather than the neocortex (which appears largely to function as a series of special purpose computers providing elaborately processed sensory information) or the brain stem (which is mainly concerned with the organisation of fixed behavioral and/or vegetative action patterns). Important exceptions to these assumptions, however, lie in those regions of the neocortex, especially in the frontal and temporal lobes, which have especially intimate connections with limbic structures; and in certain monoaminergic nuclei in the brainstem that widely innervate the limbic system.

The fifth and final assumption underlying the analysis presented here is that the major dimensions of human personality (e.g., Eysenck & Eysenck, 1969, 1976, 1985), as described by such multivariate statistical techniques as factor analysis, reflect (although not necessarily directly) individual differences in the functioning of the emotion systems of the brain.

On the basis of these assumptions, together with a considerable body of experimental data from a variety of methods of study as well as many detailed theoretical interpretations of segments of these data (Gray, 1975, 1977, 1982, 1987), it is possible, I believe, to delineate and separate three fundamental neuropsychological systems for the control of emotional behavior in the mammalian brain. Because the data on which this analysis is based are very extensive, the reader is referred to the above sources for detailed justification of the sketch map of these three systems that is offered here.

THE APPROACH SYSTEM

To a first approximation, the approach system mediates behavior elicited by reward. But this statement requires three glosses.

First, as already noted, we must distinguish between the reinforcing and eliciting properties of rewards. Thus, rewards (e.g., food, water) provide reinforcement for the acquisition and maintenance of the specific motor responses or programs that they follow. Recent experimental evidence suggests that, for at least some forms of response, this reinforcing effect of rewards may be mediated at brainstem (Huston & Borbely, 1973) and/or cerebellar (Polenchar et al., 1985) levels. But, in addition, rewards provide a general source of motivation ("incentive motivation"; Gray, 1975, chapter 5) for the performance of positively reinforced responses, a source whose intensity is proportional to the size, quality, frequency, and so on, of the reward and to the subject's proximity to it. It is likely that the mechanisms that mediate reinforcement and incentive motivation, respectively, are closely linked; but the approach system, as defined here, is concerned only with the latter.

Second, the term *reward* must be read as including relieving nonpunishment, that is, the nonoccurrence of punishment at times when the subject has some reason to expect punishment (the bottom two cells in the right hand column of Fig. 9.1). This event, when made contingent upon instrumental behavior, gives rise to active avoidance (i.e., the acquisition of new responses) as distinct from the passive avoidance (i.e., the inhibition of existing responses) that is observed when punishment is made contingent upon behavior (Fig. 9.1). There is substantial (although not conclusive) evidence that active avoidance learning is mediated and motivated by the same mechanisms that mediate learning to obtain rewards. Thus, the approach system, as defined here, is concerned with both these kinds of learning. In both cases the animal learns to approach, or produce by other means, the desired event (reward or nonpunishment): hence the term, *approach system*.

The third gloss concerns the distinction between primary and secondary reinforcers. The stimuli that elicit approach behavior are *conditioned* stimuli, which have come to be associated, probably by Pavlovian conditioning, with the primary reinforcers, be these a species of reward or nonpunishment. (In the latter case, the secondary reinforcers are often called *safety signals*.) The primary reinforcers themselves elicit a variety of fixed action patterns (e.g., eating, drinking, copulation, relaxation), depending on their exact nature. Such fixed action patterns are too specific, stimulus bound, and varied to be of central concern in the analysis of emotional behavior; correspondingly, in neural terms, they are organized at brainstem and hypothalamic levels rather than primarily in the limbic system. But note that the approach system mediates the effects of conditioned positive reinforcers once these have been established, not the conditioning process itself (although it may no doubt influence this). The basic mechanisms that give rise to Pavlovian conditioning are apparently present at many widely differing levels both of phylogeny and the neuraxis (Alkon & Farley, 1984).

With these glosses in mind, then, we may define the approach system as one that responds to conditioned rewarding and safety stimuli by facilitating behavior that maximizes further stimulation by such stimuli and the primary reinforcers with which they are associated; that is, the approach system provides incentive motivation (Gray, 1975).

It is harder to make such crisp statements when we turn to the brain. Thirty years ago, when Olds and Milner (1954) first reported that rats will electrically self-stimulate the brain, it appeared that it would take only a short time to construct a detailed map of the system that mediates the behavioral effects of rewards. However, with the passage of the years, it has become ever clearer that the interpretation of such experiments is fraught with difficulty. About the only firm statement that one can at present make is that the neural machinery corresponding to the approach system as defined here is likely to include a role for the dopaminergic projections (a) from nucleus A 10 in the ventral tegmental area to the ventral striatum (nucleus accumbens), and (b) from the substantia nigra to the dorsal striatum (Fig. 9.2; see Willner, 1985, for review). The former

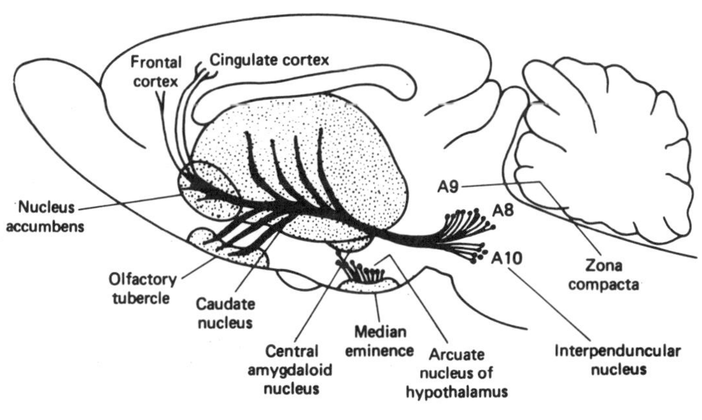

FIG. 9.2. The major dopaminergic pathways of the rat forebrain (from Cooper et al., 1982).

projection appears to relate more closely to incentive motivation as such; the latter, to the selection of the relevant motor program that is to be the beneficiary of this form of motivation. It is consistent with a major role in incentive motivation that the projection from A 10 to the nucleus accumbens has been implicated in the mediation of the hedonic and reinforcing effects of opiates and other drugs of abuse (Stewart, de Wit, and Eikelboom, 1984).

THE FIGHT/FLIGHT SYSTEM

We distinguished in the previous section between conditioned and unconditioned rewards. Similarly, we must distinguish between conditioned and unconditioned punishment. The fight/flight system mediates the behavioral effects only of unconditioned aversive events; it is the third of our systems (the behavioral inhibition system, see below) which mediates the effects of conditioned aversive stimuli. Moreover, just as we have taken *reward* to include relieving nonpunishment, so we must understand 'punishment' to include frustrative nonreward, that is, the omission or termination of reward under conditions where the subject has reason to expect reward (Fig. 9.1; Amsel, 1962). The behavior that is elicited by punishment and nonreward includes in each case components of both aggression and escape. The type of aggression observed is that qualified as *defensive* (Adams, 1979) as distinct from predatory, and the type of escape is unconditioned, consisting of a variety of fixed action patterns (running, jumping, etc.) rather than a newly learned motor skill, such as barpressing to avoid shock. Studies of the brain have demonstrated that the mechanisms that produce unconditioned escape and defensive aggression are so closely intermingled that it is often impossible to distinguish between them. For this reason, at least as a provisional tactic, it seems reasonable to postulate a single system concerned with the organization of both types of behavior rather than two separate systems. Particularly at lower brain sites mediating fight/flight behavior, there is a close relationship to mechanisms that mediate the central perception of pain (Melzack & Wall, 1983); indeed, these may well form an integral part of the fight/flight system (Graeff, 1987).

The chief brain structures that instantiate the fight/flight system are the amygdala, the ventromedial hypothalamus, and the central gray of the midbrain (Adams, 1979; de Molina & Hunsperger, 1962; Gray, 1987). These structures appear to be organized hierarchically: neurons in the ventromedial hypothalamus inhibit the final common pathway in the central gray, and neurons in the amygdala activate this pathway by disinhibition at the level of the hypothalamus (Fig. 9.3). The neural machinery mediating pain perception merges most thoroughly with the fight/flight system at the level of the central gray. At this level the fight/flight system is under three kinds of inhibition, mediated by γ-aminobutyric acid (GABA), serotonin and endogenous opiates (endorphins)

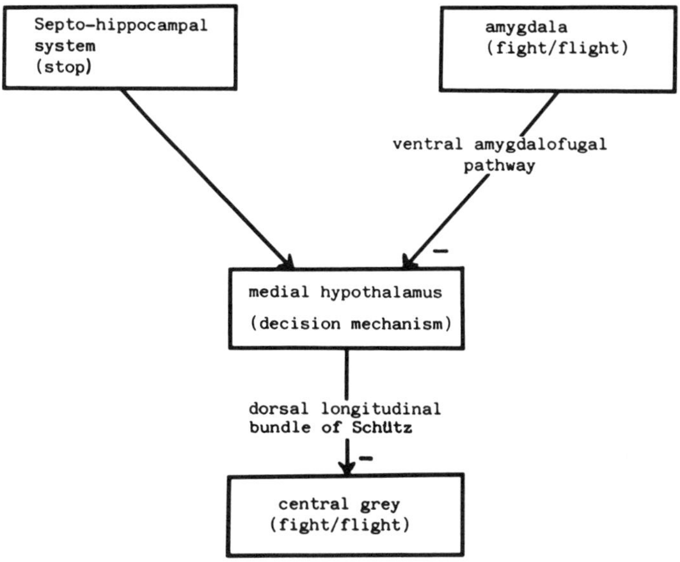

FIG. 9.3. The major components of the proposed fight/flight system. The final common pathway for fight/flight behavior is in the central grey; this is under inhibitory control from the medial hypothalamus; this inhibitory control may be disinhibited by impulses arriving from the amygdala or intensified by an input from the behavioral inhibition system (probably by way of a pathway descending from or through the lateral septal area).

respectively. Graeff (1987) has suggested that part of the clinical action of anti-anxiety drugs (including benzodiazepines, barbiturates and ethanol; Gray, 1977) is mediated by facilitation of the GABAergic inhibitory input to the central gray (these drugs are discussed more fully in the section dealing with the behavioral inhibition system). In general, however, the evidence favors an important double dissociation between the behavioral effects of anti-anxiety drugs on the one hand and opiates on the other: The former but not the latter block the effects of conditioned aversive stimuli, suggesting an action on the behavioral inhibition system; and the latter, but not the former, block the effects of unconditioned aversive stimuli, suggesting an action on the fight/flight system. This effect of opiates may be mediated by the endorphin receptors in the central gray or amygdala.

THE BEHAVIORAL INHIBITION SYSTEM

As already indicated, the behavioral inhibition system organizes responses to conditioned aversive stimuli, whether these have been formed by association with punishment or nonreward. The reactions that occur in response to such stimuli are substantially different from those that occur in response to unconditioned aversive stimuli (Gray, 1975). They are of three essential kinds (Fig. 9.4). First, all ongoing behavior is brought to a halt, although this may be only for an instant; it is this effect which motivates the term *behavioral inhibition system*. Second, there is increased attention to the environment, and especially novel features of the environment. Third, there is an increase in the level of arousal, so that the next action (which may be identical to the one interrupted by behavioral inhibition) is undertaken with increased vigor and/or speed. These same types of reaction are also seen in reponse to novel stimuli, which are also therefore deemed to act via the behavioral inhibition system (although not exclusively so; Gray et al., 1982). All three of these "outputs" of the behavioral inhibition system, to whichever input (novelty, stimuli associated with punishment, or stimuli associated with nonreward) they are a response, are blocked by all the major classes of anti-anxiety drug (Gray, 1977). For this reason, activity in the behavioral inhibition system may plausibly be deemed to constitute the human state of anxiety, as well as corresponding states in animals (Gray, 1982). This postulate has recently been supported by a number of lines of evidence from patients diagnosed as suffering from anxiety (Gray, 1988).

The major structures (Fig. 9.5; see Gray, 1982) making up the behavioral inhibition system are as follows. The centerpiece is the septohippocampal system (Elliott & Whelan, 1978); i.e., the septal area and hippocampal formation, the cholinergic projection from the medial septal nucleus and the nucleus of the diagonal band of Broca to the hippocampal formation, and the

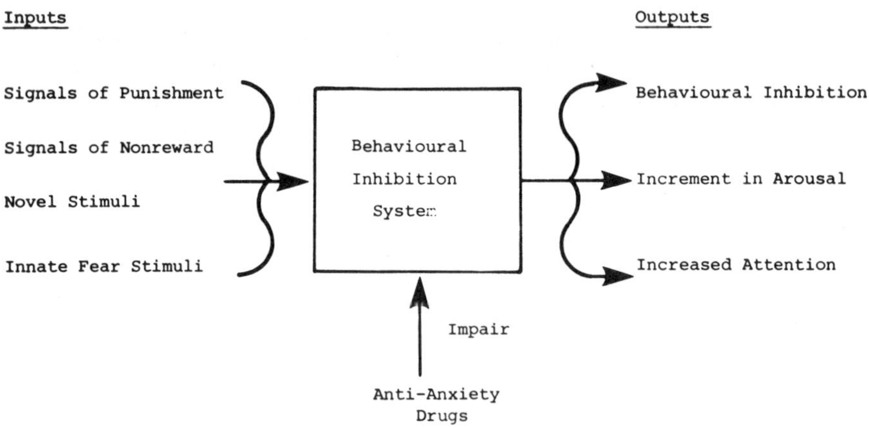

FIG. 9.4. The behavioral inhibition system. Innate fear stimuli are included among the inputs on the basis of data not discussed here. See Gray (1982, pp. 434–439).

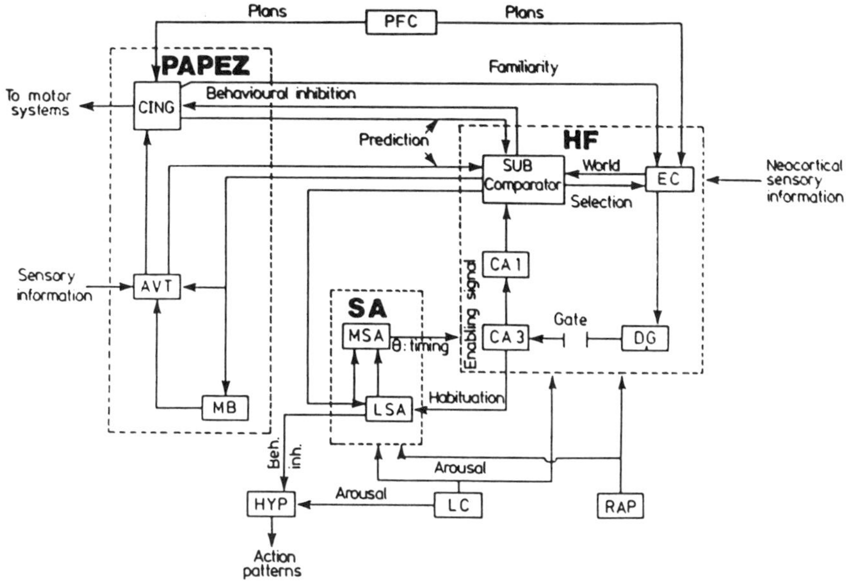

FIG. 9.5. A summary of the theory developed by Gray (1982). The three major building blocks are shown in heavy print: HF, the hippocampal formation, made up of the entorhinal cortex, EC, the dentate gyrus, DG, CA 3, CA 1, and the subicular area, SUB; SA, the septal area, containing the medial and lateral septal areas, MSA and LSA; and the Papez circuit, which receives projections from and returns them to the subicular area via the mammillary bodies, MB, anteroventral thalamus, AVT, and cingulate cortex, CING. Other structures shown are the hypothalamus, HYP, the locus coeruleus, LC, the raphe muclei, RAP, and the prefrontal cortex, PFC. Arrows show direction of projection; the projection from SUB to MSA lacks anatomical confirmation. Words in lower case show postulated functions; beh. inh., behavioral inhibition. For further explanation, see text.

return projection from the hippocampal formation to the lateral septal area. These regions receive a major neocortical input from the entorhinal cortex (in the temporal lobe); and they distribute to other regions of the brain via the subicular cortex and the Papez loop. The latter consists of a chain of connections from the subicular cortex to the mammillary bodies in the hypothalamus, from there to the anteroventral thalamus, thence to the cingulate cortex, and finally back to the subiculum. A further important neocortical projection links the prefrontal cortex to both the cingulate and the entorhinal cortex. The septohippocampal system is able to influence motor functions by way of the projection from the subiculum to the ventral striatum (Kelley & Domesick, 1982) and to the cingulate cortex; and it is able to influence hormonal processes by way of the projection from the septal area to the hypothalamus. Critical general roles are played by the ascending noradrenergic fibers from the locus coeruleus and ascending serotonergic fibers from the median raphe nucleus, which provide a diffuse input from the brainstem to the septohippocampal system, and by the ascending dopaminergic fibers from nucleus A 10 in the ventral tegmental area to the prefrontal and cingulate cortices. In addition, other noradrenergic projections (e.g., to the hypothalamus) from the locus coeruleus, and perhaps also from other brainstem noradrenergic nuclei, help mediate the "increased arousal" output of the behavioral inhibition system; and similarly, other serotonergic projections (Soubrié, 1986) (e.g., to the central gray and nucleus accumbens) from both the median and the dorsal raphe help mediate the 'behavioral inhibition' output proper. The major action of the anti-anxiety drugs upon this ramified system is probably due to enhanced GABAergic inhibition (Bowery, 1984) of activity in the ascending noradrenergic and serotonergic afferents to the septohippocampal system (Gray et al, 1984); this enhanced inhibition would have the effect of reducing the capacity of the septohippocampal system to deal with neural information entering from the entorhinal cortex (Segal, 1977a, 1977b).

The system described earlier and depicted in Fig. 9.5 is largely based on an initial analysis of the behavioral effects of the anti-anxiety drugs (Gray, 1977), followed by the attempt to identify interventions in the brain which systematically produce similar, or diametrically opposed, effects to those produced by these substances (Gray, 1982). Confidence in the reality, unity, and separate status of this system is increased by the fact that quite different lines of investigation have repeatedly homed in upon the same structures that are included in Fig. 9.5. Thus studies in which rats have been selectively bred for high or low fearfulness as measured by defecation in the open field test (Broadhurst, 1960, 1975) or for poor or good avoidance behavior (Bignami, 1965; Brush et al., 1985) have resulted in changed structure and function in the septohippocamapal system and/or the noradrenergic fibers originating in the locus coeruleus (Blizard, 1981; Drewett et al., 1977; Schwegler & Lipp, 1983; Wimer et al., 1983). Perinatal handling, which reliably alters adult levels of fearfulness (Levine, 1962), also gives rise to altered binding of glucocorticoids selectively in the prefrontal cortex and hippocampus (Meaney et al., 1985). The reliable sex differences in fearful behavior in the rat (Gray, 1979) are paralleled by differences in the electrical activity of the septohippocampal system (Drewett et al., 1977). Finally, in the monkey experiments employing electrical brain stimulation have indicated the locus coeruleus as a critical site for the integration of fearful behavior (Redmond, 1979). It is as though the system illustrated in Fig. 9.5, ramified as it is, nonetheless responds as a whole to whatever manipulations (genetic, environmental, pharmacological, etc) are employed to alter levels of fear or anxiety.

To this evidence from animal studies can now be added evidence from two recent and important studies of patients suffering from anxiety. Reiman and colleagues (1984) used the technique of positron–emission tomography (PET scanning) to compare the brains of patients prone to panic attacks to those of controls. Only one region differentiated the two groups, the one containing the entorhinal cortex (the major input to the septohippocampal system) and the subiculum (its major output). Charney and colleagues (1984) studied the response of a similar patient group to administration of a drug, yohimbine, which increases activity in the locus coeruleus. Compared to controls, the patients showed a greater biochemical reaction (measured by a metabolite of noradrenaline in plasma) to a standard dose of the drug, and also a greater rise in self-reported anxiety, these two changes being well correlated with one another. Thus, anxiety in human subjects, like analogous behavior in laboratory animals, appears to reflect activity in the septohippocampal system and in the noradrenergic fibers originating in the locus coeruleus.

In discussing the approach and fight/flight systems we considered a behavioral and a neural level of analysis. The data base relating to the behavioral inhibition system is more extensive than for either of these other two systems, so permitting us to make the transition to a third, equally necessary level of analysis, that of information processing (or cognition). In speculating about the cognitive functions discharged by the neural system depicted in Fig. 9.5, I have proposed (Gray, 1982) that it plays a general monitoring role in checking that behavior goes according to plan. To this end the system generates predictions (instant by instant, at a rate of about ten times a second) as to the next most likely event. In doing so, it draws upon stored information (perhaps located in the neocortex of the temporal lobes) concerning past regularities (stimulus–stimulus or response—stimulus, generated by the processes of classical and instrumental conditioning respectively), together with information describing the current state of the animal's "world" (entering via the entorhinal cortex) and the animal's current motor program (derived from the prefrontal cortex). The system then compares predicted with actual events. If things go according to plan (that is, predictions match actual events), the system continues to operate simply in "checking mode," behavior remaining under the control of other, unspecified "brain systems." If, however, there is a mismatch (novelty, that is, an unpredicted event occurs or a predicted event fails to occur), or if the next predicted event is aversive (i.e., punishment or nonreward, or a stimulus associated with these primary reinforcers), the system switches to "control mode," taking direct control over behavior and operating the outputs of the behavioral inhibition system as shown in Fig. 9.4 (i.e., inhibition of ongoing behavior, increased attention, and increased arousal). Detailed proposals as to the neural machinery which carries out each of these functions can be found in Gray (1982); see also Fig. 9.5.

These cognitive functions can be mapped onto the chief clinical phenomena of human anxiety by the suppositions that phobic behavior largely represents the behavioral inhibition output of the behavioral inhibition system when it is in control mode, and that obsessional symptoms reflect excessive checking when the system is in checking mode. Certain clinical phenomena, however, require the further postulate that, in humans, the ascending monoaminergic control over the septohippocampal system is supplemented by a descending control via the projection from the prefrontal to the entorhinal cortex, allowing neocortical language systems to generate anxiety to verbally coded material. The autonomic symptoms of anxiety are in part probably mediated by noradrenergic fibers descending from the locus coeruleus into the spinal cord (Redmond, 1979, but see the discussion of interactions between the behavioral inhibition and fight/flight systems later).

This is, of course, a highly condensed version of a complex neuropsychological theory. For further details the reader is referred to Gray (1982, 1987) and Gray and Rawlins (1986).

INTERACTIONS BETWEEN SYSTEMS

Although it is my contention that each of the systems described previously is to an important degree separate from all the other systems that make up the great overall system that is the brain, nonetheless it is clear that they can only discharge their functions by interacting with the rest of the brain, and in particular with each other. As in the case of the individual systems, we can consider such interactions from both a behavioral and a neurological point of view.

Behaviorally, the very specification of the behavioral inhibition system requires that it should be able to inhibit activity in each of the other two systems. There is indeed a wealth of evidence that the behavioral inhibition system is able to inhibit approach behavior (whether to stimuli associated with reward or to stimuli associated with nonpunishment), and rather less evidence that it can inhibit reactions to unconditioned punishment. In the latter case the inhibition appears to include the pain sensation itself. Thus, presentation to an animal in pain of a stimulus previously associated with foot shock reduces behavioral responses to the stimulus eliciting pain; this effect can be reversed by administration of opiate antagonists, such as naloxone, so it is presumably mediated by endorphin receptors (Bolles & Fanselow, 1980; Fanselow & Baackes, 1982; Gray, 1987). In addition to these effects of the behavioral inhibition system upon the activities of the other two systems, certain phenomena observed in conflict situations (Gray, 1987; Gray & Smith, 1969) strongly suggest that the approach system can inhibit the behavioral inhibition system (Fig. 9.6).

The most likely sites of interaction between the behavioral inhibition and approach systems lie in the ventral striatum and lateral septal area (Fig. 9.7). As we have seen, the dopaminergic input from nucleus A 10 in the ventral tegmental area to the nucleus accumbens in the ventral striatum (Fig. 9. 2) is the best candidate for the neural instantiation of incentive motivation. It is intriguing, therefore, that the ventral striatum is also a major target for fibers directed from the subicular area (Kelley & Domesick, 1982), which provides the main output from the septohippocampal system. The ventral striatum, then, is an ideal site at which the behavioral inhibition system could inhibit striatal output destined to facilitate motor behavior aimed at the attainment of reward or nonpunishment. The reverse interaction perhaps takes place in the lateral septal area. This region too is the recipient of dopaminergic afferents from A 10, as well

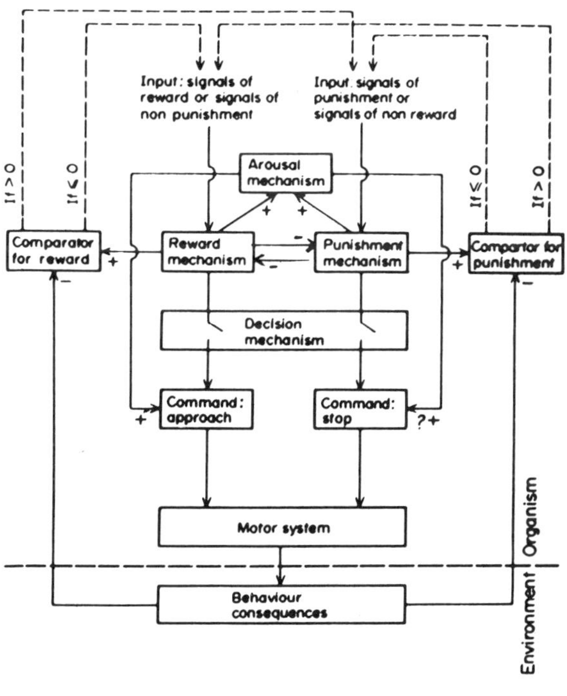

FIG. 9.6. The Gray and Smith (1969) Model. Dashed lines indicated inputs which occur on trial n + 1 as a result of classical conditioning of exteroceptive, interoceptive or proprioceptive CSs to the consequences of behavior on trial n. +, excitation; −, inhibition.

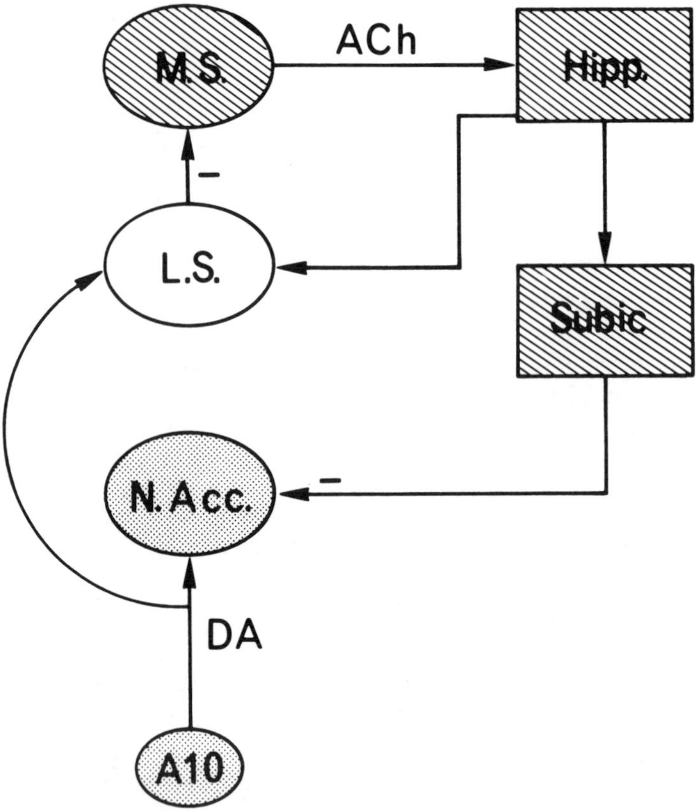

FIG. 9.7. A possible neural substrate for the type of interaction between the approach (reward) and behavioral inhibition (punishment) systems depicted in FIG. 9.6. M.S., medial septal area, origin of a cholinergic (ACh) projection to the hippocampal formation (Hipp.), which in turn projects to the lateral septal area (L.S.) and the subicular area (Subic). These structures form part of the behavioral inhibition system. The approach system includes the dopaminergic (DA) projection from nucleus A 10 in the ventral tegmental area to the nucleus accumbens (N. Acc.). The subicular projection to the nucleus accumbens may mediate inhibition (−) of the approach system; and the projection from A 10 to the lateral septal area, together with the projection from there to the medial septal area, may mediate the reciprocal inhibitory link from the approach to the behavioral inhibition system.

as a projection from the hippocampus. Furthermore, recent work from Jaffard's laboratory (Galey et al., 1985) has shown that the dopaminergic fibers exercise inhibitory control over the major cholinergic projection from the medial septal area to the hippocampal formation. Thus, in an approach–avoidance conflict

(Miller, 1959), the outcome would perhaps be determined by (a) the balance between the dopaminergic and subicular inputs to the ventral striatum, coupled with (b) the balance between the dopaminergic and hippocampal projections to the lateral septal area.

There are at least three ways in which the behavioral inhibition system can exert inhibitory control over the fight/flight system.

First, there is a descending pathway from the lateral septal area to the ventromedial hypothalamus (Albert & Chew, 1980). Rather than exerting simple inhibitory control over fight/flight behavior, it is possible that this route switches dominant aggression to submissive behavior depending on social rank (Adams, 1979).

Second, as previously noted, neurons in the central gray are under inhibitory serotonergic control. Graeff (1987), who has used a variety of stimulation and pharmacological techniques in an intensive study of this region of the brain, has suggested: (a) that serotonergic inhibition of the central gray plays an important role in controlling the strong autonomic discharge that accompanies fight/flight behavior; and (b) that it is a phasic failure in such control that gives rise to panic attacks in the human syndromes of anxiety state and agoraphobia. Such attacks do not typically respond to medication with anti-anxiety drugs; they do, however, respond to antidepressants with serotonin-uptake blocking activity (Klein et al., 1985). Graeff (1987) has proposed that the latter effect is due to enhancement of serotonergic inhibition over the central gray neurons responsible for autonomic outflow. If this analysis is correct, it implies that panic attacks characterize patients who chronically experience intense activity in both the fight/flight and behavioral inhibition systems, and that the attacks actually take place when the inhibition exerted by the latter system upon the former temporarily fails.

The third route by which the behavioral inhibition system can inhibit the fight/flight system includes passage via an endorphin receptor: as noted earlier, inhibition of pain by conditioned aversive stimuli can be blocked by opiate antagonists (Fanselow & Baackes, 1982). It is possible that the relevant opiate receptors are those located in the central gray. At this level of the fight/flight system, as also in the spinal cord, there appears to be close coordination between endorphinergic and serotonergic neurons in the inhibition of pain (Melzack & Wall, 1983). Another possibility (not exclusive of the former) consists in the dense population of opiate receptors found in the amygdala.

A final form of interaction between the behavioral inhibition system and the other two is excitatory rather than inhibitory. This type of interaction is implicit in the description given previously of the arousal output of the behavioral inhibition system. This seems to prepare the animal for especially vigorous action when action next becomes possible. This function of the behavioral inhibition system is apparently mediated largely by noradrenergic fibers, mainly those originating in the locus coeruleus (Redmond, 1979). These fibers innervate target organs that are widely distributed throughout the brain (Fig. 9.8), and appear in general to facilitate the reaction of these targets to afferents arriving from other sources. In the hippocampal formation, for example, the noradrenergic input facilitates the response of hippocampal neurons to stimuli arriving along the perforant path from the entorhinal cortex (Segal, 1977a, 1977b; Fig. 9.5). An action of this kind could prime approach, fight/flight or appetitive consummatory behavior, depending on the functions discharged by the relevant target organ (Fig. 9.8 and 9.9). In accordance with this analysis, anxiogenic stimuli increase noradrenergic activity throughout the brain; and this effect is blocked by administration of anti-anxiety drugs (Lidbrink et al., 1973; Redmond, 1979).

These various interactions between the behavioral inhibition system and the other two systems are summarized in Fig. 9.9.

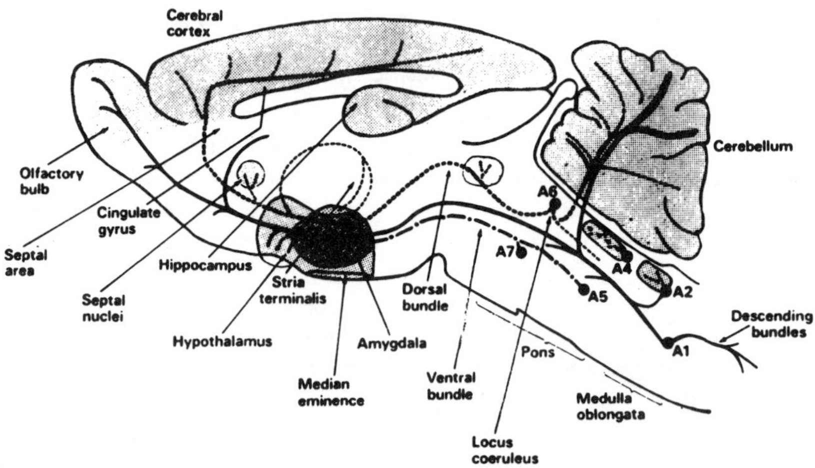

FIG. 9.8. Sagittal representation of the rat brain, showing the principal ascending and descending noradreneric pathways. Cell bodies in the locus coeruleus (A6) give rise to pathways (---) innervating all cortical areas of the brain. The dorsal bundle arising from A6 also innervates areas of the amygdala and anterior hypothalamus, while a short descending pathway innervates lower brainstem nuclei. Cell group A1 (______) gives rise to a descending bulbo-spinal pathway, and a major ascending ventral pathway, which follows the course of the medial forebrain bundle all the way to the olfactory bulb. This ventral bundle, which comprises ascending fibres from cell groups A5 and A7 (-.-.-) as well as from A1 and A2, gives off branches to the lateral mammillary nuclei, the lateral and ventral hypothalamus (the latter providing terminals to the median eminence and infundibulum), and to large parts of the limbic forebrain (including the anterior medial amygdaloid complex, the ventral medial septum, and cingulum). Shaded areas indicate regions of noradrenergic terminals (from Livett 1973).

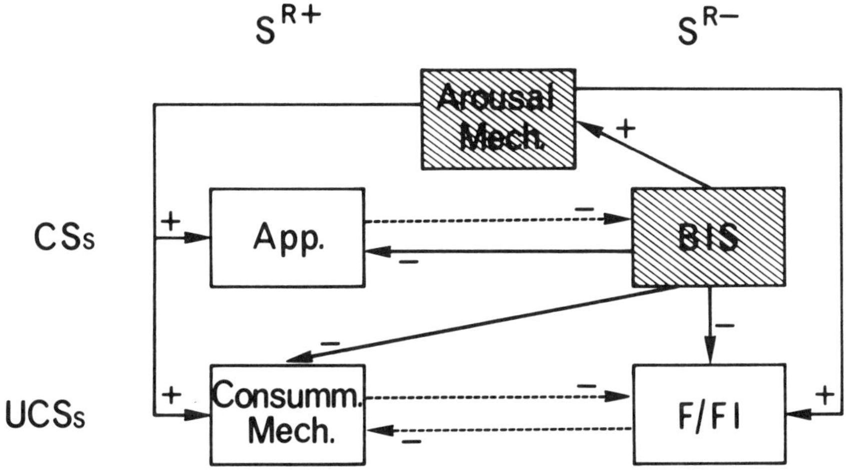

FIG. 9.9. Interactions between the Behavioral Inhibition System (BIS) and its associated Arousal Mechanism with the Approach (App.) and Fight/Flight (F/F1) Systems and Consummatory Mechanisms for fixed action patterns. Systems on the left respond to positive reinforcers (S^{R+}),those on the right to negative reinforcers or punishers (S^{R-}). Systems in the upper row respond to conditioned reinforcers (CSs), those in the lower row to unconditioned reinforcers (UCSs). +, excitation; −, inhibition.

PERSONALITY

As noted at the start of the chapter, the approach adopted here assumes that the major dimensions of human personality reflect consistent patterns of individual differences in the functioning of separate emotion systems in the brain (Gray, 1968). Ideally, therefore, in the description of personality dimensions one would focus on behavior patterns likely to reflect the activities of each of the three neuropsychological systems delineated earlier. However, a vast volume of research has gone into the construction of existing personality descriptions, which cannot therefore lightly be thrown aside. In any case, these descriptions, and especially the one developed by the Eysencks (1969, 1976, 1983), provide convenient and useful frameworks within which one can situate different diagnostic groups and psychiatric conditions. These descriptions of personality have relied heavily upon the methods of multivariate statistics, and especially factor analysis. This technique can establish how many independent dimensions of variation there are in a given data set, but it cannot fix the location of these dimensions in any nonarbitrary way (Gray, 1981). The system developed by the Eysencks has three independent dimensions (introversion–extraversion, neuroticism, and psychoticism). The recurrence of the number three may indicate no more than coincidence with the number of emotion systems we have distinguished above. Nonetheless, it suggests the possibility that the three Eysenckian dimensions reflect (no doubt indirectly and with some distortion) the activities of these very same systems (Gray, 1972). If so, we might light upon dimensions that map more directly upon our three brain systems by the simple expedient of rotating the Eysenckian factors into new (but still mutually orthogonal) positions within the same overall three-dimensional space.

Within the more tractable two-dimensional space bounded by the axes of introversion–extraversion and neuroticism, I have proposed a rotation of this kind before, giving rise to one dimension (trait anxiety) that directly reflects individual differences in the reactivity of the behavioral inhibition system, and to a second (impulsivity) which similarly reflects dthe reactivity of the approach system (Gray, 1970). The resulting diagram (Fig. 9.10) shows that one can then treat introversion–extraversion as a derived dimension, reflecting the balance between the reactivities of the behavioral inhibition and approach systems.

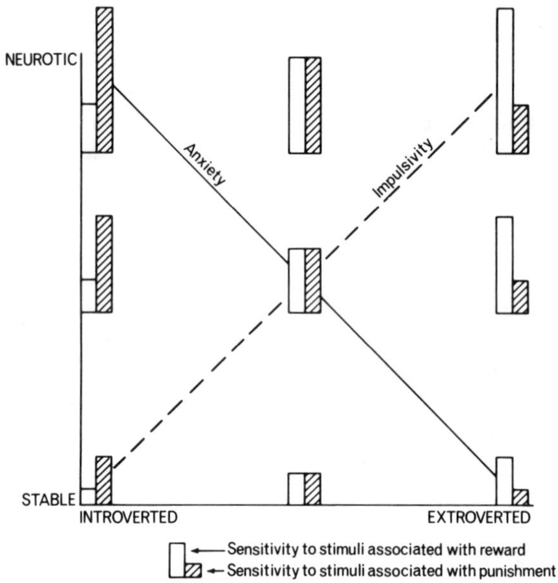

FIG. 9.10. Rotation of Eysenck's dimensions of neuroticism and introversion-extraversion proposed by Gray (1970). The dimension of trait Anxiety represents the steepest rate of growth in susceptibility to signals of punishment (and other adequate inputs to the behavioral inhibition system); the dimension of Impulsivity represents the steepest rate of growth in susceptibility to signals of reward. Introversion–extraversion now becomes a derived dimension, reflecting the balance of susceptibility to signals of punishment and reward, respectively; and neuroticism similarly reflects the sum of these two types of susceptibility to signals of reinforcement.

Given our discussion of interactions between these two systems (Fig. 9.6), this notion of balance may itself have a concrete neurological instantiation, in the form of the various inputs to the ventral striatum and lateral septal area illustrated in Fig. 9.7. Figure 9.10 also suggests that one may similarly treat neuroticism as a derived dimension, reflecting a summation of the reactivities of the behavioral inhibition and approach systems. This notion may have a less unified neurological reality than the corresponding treatment of introversion–extraversion. However, one can perhaps make out the case that a summation between the (primarily dopaminergic) activity making up incentive motivation (Fig. 9.2) and the noradrenergic activity that constitutes the arousal output of the behavioral inhibition system (Fig. 9.8 and 9.9) could underlie neuroticism.

A diagram similar in principle to that of Fig. 9.10 can be constructed using the behavioral inhibition system and, in place of the approach system, the fight/flight system. Such a diagram is presented in Fig. 9.11. There are no good names at present for a dimension reflecting individual differences in the reactivity of the fight/flight system; although the Eysenckian axis of psychoticism, (Eysenck & Eysenck, 1976) has some claim to constituting such a dimension

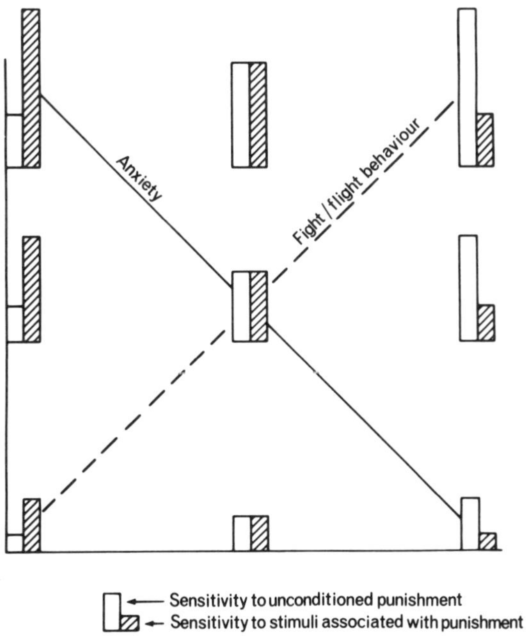

FIG. 9.11. Possible relations between individual differences in the susceptibility to anxiety and to the display of fight/flight behavior, along similar lines to those illustrated in Fig. 9.10.

(Gray, 1972). Given our previous discussion of likely interactions between the behavioral inhibition and fight/flight systems, there is some reason to consider both the balance between, and the summation of, the reactivities of these two systems as possessing their own neurological reality. If, for example, Graeff (1987; see earlier) is correct in his speculations concerning the role of the central gray in determining the symptoms and course of panic attacks, we might see the occurrence of such attacks as depending on the momentary balance between the behavioral inhibition and fight/flight systems; and the individuals who are prone to them, as having chronically high reactivity in both systems.

One can obviously use the approach and fight/flight systems to construct yet a third two-dimensional diagram (not to mention the three-dimensional diagram that one obtains by putting all three systems together simultaneously; see Gray, 1983, for one attempt along these lines). But I desist from playing what is still at present an amusing game. It will cease to be a game if and when we are able to situate with confidence relevant diagnostic categories, whether among adults or children, at appropriate points in the space that houses these speculations.

REFERENCES

Adams, D. B. (1979). Brain mechanisms for offence, defense, and submission. *The Behavioral & Brain Sciences 2*, 201–241.

Albert, D. J., & Chew, G. L. (1980). The septal forebrain and the inhibitory modulation of attack and defence in the rat: a review. *Behavioral and Neural Biology, 30*, 357–388.

Alkon, D., & Farley, J. (Eds.). (1984). *Primary neural substrates of learning and behavioral change*. Cambridge: Cambridge University Press.

Amsel, A. (1962). Frustrative nonreward in partial reinforcement and discrimination learning: some recent history and a theoretical extension. *Psychological Review*, 69, 306–328.

Bignami, G. (1965). Selection for high rates and low rates of avoidance conditioning in the rat. *Animal Behaviour, 13*, 221–227.

Blizard, D. A. (1981) The Maudsley reactive and nonreactive strains: a North American perspective. *Behavioral Genetics, 11*, 469–489.

Bolles, R. C., & Fanselow, M. S. (1980). A perceptual defensive-recuperative model of fear and pain. *The Behavioral & Brain Sciences*, 3, 291–323.

Bowery, N. G. (Ed.). (1984). *Actions and interactions of* GABA *and benzodiazepines*. New York: Raven Press.

Broadhurst, P. L. (1960). Application of biometrical genetics to the inheritance of behaviour. In H. J. Eysenck (Ed.), *Experiments in personality* (Vol. 1, pp. 3–102). London: Routledge & Kegan Paul.

Broadhurst, P. L. (1975).The Maudsley reactive and nonreactive strains of rats: A survey. *Behavioral Genetics*, 5, 299–319.

Brush, F. R., Baron, S., Forehlich, J. C., Ison, J. R., Pellegrino, L. J., Philips, D. S., Sakellanis, R. C., & Williams, V. N. (1985). Genetic differences in avoidance learning by *Rattus norvegicus:* Escape/avoidance responding, sensitivity to electric shock, discrimination learning, and open-field behavior. *Journal of Comparative Psychology,* 99, 60–73.

Charney, D. S., Heininger, G. R., & Breier, A. (1984). Noradrenergic function in panic anxiety. *Archives of General Psychiatry, 41,* 751–763.

Cooper, J. R., Bloom, F. E., & Roth, R. H. (1982). *The biochemical basis of neuropharmacology* (4th ed.). New York: Oxford University Press.

de Molina, F. A., & Hunsperger, R. W. (1962). Organisation of the subcortical system governing defence and flight reactions in the cat. *Journal of Physiology, 160,* 200–213.

Drewett, R. F., Gray, J. A., James, D. T. D., McNaughton, N., Valero, I., & Dudderidge, H. J. (1977). Sex and strain differences in septal driving of the hippocampal theta rhythm as a function of frequency: effects of gonadectomy and gonadal hormones. *Neuroscience, 2,* 1033–1041.

Elliott, K., & Whelan, J. (Eds.). (1978). Functions of the septo-hippocampal system. *Ciba Foundation Symposium 58 (New Series).* Amsterdam: Elsevier.

Eysenck, H. J., & Eysenck, M. W. (1985). *Personality and individual differences: A natural science approach.* New York: Plenum Press.

Eysenck, H. J., & Eysenck, S. B. G. (1969). *Personality structure and measurement.* London: Routledge & Kegan Paul.

Eysenck, S. B. G., & Eysenck, H. J. (1976). *Psychoticism as a dimension of personality.* London: Hodder and Stoughton.

Fanselow, M. S., & Baackes, M. P. (1982). Conditioned fear-induced opiate analgesia on the formalin test: evidence for two aversive motivational systems. *Learning and Motivation, 13,* 200–221.

Galey, D., Durkin, T., Sitakis, G., Kempf, E., & Jaffard, R. (1975). Facilitation of spontaneous and learned spatial behaviours following 6-hydroxydopamine lesions of the lateral septum: a cholinergic hypothesis. *Brain Research, 340,* 171–174.

Graeff, F. G. (1987). The anti-aversive action of drugs. In T. Thompson, P. B. Dews, & J. Barrett (Eds.), *Advances in behavioral pharmacology* (Vol. 5, pp. 129–156). Hillsdale, NJ: Lawrence Erlbaum Associates.

Gray, J. A. (1968). The Lister lecture. The physiological basis of personality. *Advancement of Science, 24,* 293–305.

Gray, J. A. (1970). The psychophysiological basis of introversion-extraversion. *Behaviour Research and Therapy, 8,* 249–266.

Gray, J. A. (1972). Causal theories of personality and how to test them. In J. R. Royce (Ed.), *Multivariate analysis and psychological theory* (pp. 409–463). London: Academic Press.

Gray, J. A. (1975). *Elements of a two-process theory of learning.* London: Academic Press.

Gray, J. A. (1977). Drug effects on fear and frustration: possible limbic site of action of minor tranquilizers. In L. L. Iversen, S. D. Iversen, & S. H. Snyder (Eds.), *Handbook of psychopharmacology* (Vol. 8, pp. 433–529). New York: Plenum.

Gray, J. A. (1979). Emotionality in male and female rodents: a reply to Archer. *British Journal of Psychology, 70,* 425–440.

Gray, J. A. (1981). A critique of Eysenck's theory of personality. In H. J. Eysenck (Ed.), *A model for personality* (pp. 246–276). Berlin: Springer.

Gray, J. A. (1982). *The neuropsychology of anxiety: An enquiry into the functions of the septo–hippocampal system*. Oxford: Oxford University Press.

Gray, J. A. (1983). Where should we search for biologically based dimensions of personality? *Zeitschrift für Differentielle und Diagnostische Psychologie, 4,* 165–176.

Gray, J. A. (1987). *The psychology of fear and stress* (2nd ed.). Cambridge: Cambridge University Press.

Gray, J. A. (1988). Anxiety and personality. In M. Roth, G. D. Burrows, & R. Noyes (Eds.), *Handbook of anxiety*, Vol. 1, pp. 231–257. Amsterdam: Elsevier.

Gray, J. A. (in press). Neural systems, emotion and personality. In J. Madden, S. Matthysse, & J. Barchas (Eds.), *Adaptation, learning and affect*. New York: Raven Press.

Gray, J. A., Quintero, S., Mellanby, J., Buckland, C., Fillenz, M., & Fung, S. C. (1984). Some biochemical, behavioural and electrophysiological tests of the GABA hypothesis of anti–anxiety drug action. In N. G. Bowery (Ed.), *Actions and interactions of GABA and benzodiazepines* (pp. 239–262). New York: Raven Press.

Gray, J. A., & Rawlins, J. N. P. (1986). Comparator and buffer memory: an attempt to integrate two models of hippocampal function. In R. L. Isaacson & K. H. Pribram (Eds.), *The hippocampus* (Vol. 4, pp. 159–201). New York: Plenum Press.

Gray, J. A., & Smith, P. T. (1969). An arousal-decision model for partial reinforcement and discrimination learning. In R. Gilbert & N. S. Sutherland (Eds.), *Animal discrimination learning* (pp. 243–272). London: Academic Press.

Hebb, D. O. (1955). Drives and the C.N.S. (conceptual nervous system). *Psychological Review, 62,* 243–254.

Huston, J. P., & Borbely, A. A. (1973). Operant conditioning in forebrain ablated rats by use of rewarding hypothalamic stimulation. *Brain Research, 50,* 467–472.

Kelley, A.E., & Domesick, V. B. (1982). The distribution of the projection from the hippocampal formation to the nucleus accumbens in the rat: an anterograde– and retrograde–horseradish peroxidase study. *Neuroscience, 7,* 2321–2335.

Klein, D. F., Rabkin, J. G., & Gorman, J. M. (1985). Ethological and pathophysiological inferences from the pharmacological treatment of anxiety. In A. H. Tuma & J. D. Maser (Eds.), *Anxiety and the anxiety disorders* (pp. 501–532). Hillsdale, NJ: Lawrence Erlbaum Associates.

Levine, S. (1962). Psychophysiological effects of infantile stimulation. In E. L. Bliss (Ed.), *Roots of behavior* (pp. 246–253). New York: Harper.

Lidbrink, P., Corrodi, H., Fuxe, K., & Olson, L. (1973). The effects of benzodiazepines, meprobamate, and barbiturates on central monoamine neurons. In S. Garattini, E. Mussini, & L. O. Randall (Eds.), *The benzodiazepines* (pp. 203–223). New York: Raven Press.

Livett, B. G. (1973). Histochemical visualization of peripheral and central adrenergic neurones. In L. L. Iversen (Ed.), *Catecholamines* (British Medical Bulletin Suppl. 29, 93–99).

Meany, M. J., Aitken, D. H., Bodnoff, S. R., Ing, C. J., Tatarewicz, J. E., & Sapolsky, R. M. (1985). Early postnatal handling alters glucocorticoid receptor concentrations in selected brain regions. *Behavioral Neuroscience, 99,* 765–770.

Melzack, R., & Wall, P. D. (1983). *The challenge of pain*. New York: Basic Books.

Miller, N. E. (1959). Liberalization of basic S-R concepts: Extensions to conflict behavior, motivation and social learning. In S. Koch (Ed.), *Psychology: A study of a science* (study 1, Vol. 2, pp. 196–292). New York: McGraw-Hill.

Olds, J., & Milner, P. (1954). Positive reinforcement produced by electrical stimulation of septal area and other regions. *Journal of Comparative and Physiological Psychology, 47*, 419–427.

Polenchar, B. E., Patterson, M. M., Lavond, D. G., & Thompson, R. F. (1985). Cerebellar lesions abolish an avoidance response in rabbits. *Behavioral and Neural Biology, 44*, 221–227.

Redmond, D. E., Jr. (1979). New and old evidence for the involvement of a brain norepinephrine system in anxiety. In W. G. Fann, I. Karacan, A. D. Pokorny, & R. L. Williams (Eds.), *Phenomenology and treatment of anxiety* (pp. 153–203). New York: Spectrum.

Reiman, E. M., Raichle, M. E., Butler, F. K., Hersovitch, P., & Robins, E. (1984). A focal brain abnormality in panic disorder, a severe form of anxiety. *Nature, 310*, 683–685.

Schwegler, H., & Lipp, H. P. (1983). Hereditary covariatons of neuronal circuitry and behavior: Correlations between the proportions of hippocampal synaptic fields in the regio inferior and two-way avoidance in mice and rats. *Behavioral and Brain Research, 7*, 1–38.

Segal, M. (1977a). The effects of brainstem priming stimulation on interhemispheric hippocampal responses in the awake rat. *Experimental Brain Research, 28*, 529–541.

Segal, M. (1977b). Excitability changes in rat hippocampus during conditioning. *Experimental Brain Research, 55*, 67–73.

Soubrié, P. (1986). Reconciling the role of central serotonin neurons in human and animal behavior. *The Behavioral and Brain Sciences*, 9, 319–364.

Stewart, J., de Wit, H., & Eikelboom, R. (1984). Role of unconditioned and conditioned drug effects in the self-administration of opiates and stimulants. *Psychological Review, 91*, 251–268.

Willner, P. (1985). *Depression: A psychobiological synthesis*. New York: Wiley.

Wimer, C., Wimer, R., & Wimer, J. (1983). An association between granule cell density in the dentate gyrus and two–way avoidance conditioning in the house mouse. *Behavioral Neuroscience, 97*, 844–856.

Author Index

Numbers in *italics* denote complete reference citation.

T

Subject Index